NURSES AND FAMILIES
A Guide to Family Assessment and Intervention

Second Edition

LORRAINE M. WRIGHT, RN, PhD
Director, Family Nursing Unit
Professor, Faculty of Nursing
University of Calgary
Calgary, Alberta, Canada

MAUREEN LEAHEY, RN, PhD
Director, Outpatient Mental Health Program
Calgary District Hospital Group
Adjunct Associate Professor
Faculties of Nursing and Medicine (Psychiatry)
University of Calgary
Calgary, Alberta, Canada

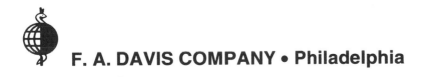

F. A. DAVIS COMPANY • Philadelphia

F. A. Davis Company
1915 Arch Street
Philadelphia, PA 19103

Printed in Canada

Last digit indicates print number: 10 9 8

Publisher, Nursing: Robert G. Martone
Production Editor: Crystal S. McNichol
Cover Design By: Steven R. Morrone

As new scientific information becomes available through basic and clinical research, recommended treatments and drug therapies undergo changes. The author(s) and publisher have done everything possible to make this book accurate, up to date, and in accord with accepted standards at the time of publication. The authors, editors, and publisher are not responsible for errors or omissions or for consequences from application of the book and make no warranty, expressed or implied, in regard to the contents of the book. Any practice described in this book should be applied by the reader in accordance with professional standards of care used in regard to the unique circumstances that may apply in each situation. The reader is advised always to check product information (package inserts) for changes and new information regarding dose and contraindications before administering any drug. Caution is especially urged when using new or infrequently ordered drugs.

Library of Congress Cataloging-in-Publication Data

Wright, Lorraine M., 1944–
    Nurses and families : a guide to family assessment and intervention / Lorraine M. Wright, Maureen Leahey. —2nd ed.
      p. cm.
    Includes bibliographical references and index.
    ISBN 0–8036–9605–1 (soft cover : alk. paper)
    1. Family nursing. 2. Family assessment. I. Leahey, Maureen, 1944– . II. Title.
    [DNLM: 1. Family Health—nurses' instruction. 2. Interviews—methods—nurses' instruction. 3. Nursing Assessment. WY 100 W951n 1994]
    RT120.F34W75 1994
    610.73—dc20
    DNLM/DLC
    for Library of Congress
                                                                   93–43430
                                                                    CIP

To Wendy L. Watson for high-spirited friendship, synergistic colleagueship, and years and years of believing in me.

Lorraine M. Wright

and

To Nora Sheehan Neus, my mother, who cared so deeply.

Maureen Leahey

PREFACE

Nurses are renowned for providing holistic healthcare to individuals in all types of clinical settings. Also respected but less well known is the healthcare that nurses provide for families. Despite the fact that 10 years have elapsed since the publication of the first edition of this book, nurses have received little acclaim for their work with families. This second edition is written in recognition of the family work nurses already do and of nurses' desires to increase their involvement with families in healthcare.

Most nurses have a "family mindedness," and some have been taught a conceptual base for family work. Many, however, struggle with how to apply their conceptual framework in actual clinical practice. What they desire are ways to enhance their interviewing skills so that they can engage, assess, and intervene effectively with families, not just with individuals.

This thoroughly revised second edition of *Nurses and Families* is an ideal "how-to" basic text for undergraduate, graduate, and practicing nurses. It is the only textbook on the market that provides specific how-to guidelines for family assessment and intervention. The practical how-to guide for clinical work offers the opportunity for nursing students, practitioners, and educators to deliver better healthcare to families. Students and practitioners of community health nursing, parent-child nursing, pediatrics, mental health nursing, and gerontic nursing will find it most useful. Nurse educators who presently teach a family-centered approach and those who will be introducing the concept of the "family as the patient" will find it a valuable resource. Educators involved in continuing education courses will be able to use this book to update nurses' clinical skills in family-centered care.

Nurses and Families provides specific guidelines for nurses to consider when preparing for, conducting, and documenting family meetings from the first interview through to discharge. Actual clinical case examples are extensively given throughout the book. These case examples reflect ethnic diversity and various family developmental life cycle stages. Issues in a variety of practice settings are addressed. The clinical practice ideas are based on solid theory, research, and the authors' own extensive clinical experience with families.

The major purposes of this book are to (1) provide nurses with a sound theoretical foundation for family assessment and intervention; (2) provide nurses with clear, concise, and comprehensive family assessment and intervention models; (3) provide a guideline for beginning family interviewing skills; and (4) give detailed ideas and suggestions with clinical examples of how to prepare, conduct, and document family interviews.

In this second edition the following features are unique:

1. The Calgary Family Assessment Model (CFAM) has been thoroughly updated and revised. It is easy to apply, practical, and relevant for busy nurses.
2. The Calgary Family Intervention Model (CFIM) is introduced. It is the first family intervention model for nurses by nurses and offers interventions to assist with cognitive, affective, and behavioral family functioning.
3. The family developmental life cycle has been expanded to include divorce and postdivorce life cycles, remarried family life cycle, adoptive family life cycle, and a comparison of professional with low-income family life cycles. The range of family forms in society today is reflected.

The first five chapters provide the conceptual base for working with families. To be able to interview families and accurately identify strengths and intervene with a problem, it is first necessary to have a sound conceptual framework.

Chapter 1 establishes a rationale for family assessment and intervention. It describes the conceptual shift involved in considering the family system, rather than the individual, as the unit of healthcare. It outlines the indications and contraindications for family assessment and intervention. As well, an overview of the family intervention literature is presented.

Chapter 2 addresses the major concepts of systems, cybernetics, communication, and change theory. Clinical examples of the application of these concepts are given.

Chapter 3 presents the CFAM, a comprehensive, three-pronged, structural, developmental, and functional family-assessment framework. This widely adopted model has been thoroughly updated and revised to reflect the current range of family forms in North American society. Specific questions that the nurse may ask the family are provided. Two structural assessment tools are delineated, and instructions are given for how to use them in interviewing families. Excerpts from actual family interviews are presented to illustrate how to use the model in clinical practice.

Chapter 4 introduces the CFIM, taking the nurse beyond assessment and presenting interventions to perturb change in the cognitive, affective, and behavioral domains of family functioning. Actual clinical examples of family work are presented, and a variety of interventions are offered for consideration. Nurses traditionally have focused only on assessment with families because there have not been family intervention models within nursing to draw on. CFIM corrects this omission.

Chapter 5 delineates the competencies and perceptual, conceptual, and executive skills necessary for family assessment and intervention. The skills are written in the form of training objectives, and clinical examples are given to help broaden the nurse's understanding of how to use these skills. Nurse educators, in particular, may find this chapter useful in focusing their evaluation of students' family interviewing skills.

The specific how-to section of the book is included in Chapters 6 through 9. The absence of ideas on how to prepare, conduct, and document family interviews is frequently the greatest inhibitor to offering more family-oriented healthcare. Thus, Chapter 6 presents guidelines useful when preparing for family interviews. Ideas are given for developing hypotheses, choosing an appropriate interview setting, and making the first telephone contact with the family.

Chapter 7 delineates the various stages of the first interview and the remaining stages of the entire interviewing process: engagement, assessment, intervention, and termination. Actual clinical case examples illustrate the practice of conducting the interviews.

Chapter 8 offers ideas on how to document in a manageable fashion the vast amounts of data generated during family assessment and intervention meetings. Suggestions are given for how to develop a strength and problems list, assessment summary, progress record, and discharge synopsis.

Chapter 9 highlights how to terminate with families in a therapeutic manner. Ideas are given for family-initiated and nurse-initiated termination as well as for discharges determined by the healthcare system.

The major difference between this book and other books focused on the nursing of families is that this book's primary emphasis in on *how to* interview families. We wish to emphasize, however, that this book does not offer a "cook book" approach to family interviewing. The real development of skills results from actual clinical practice and supervisory feedback. We envision this book as a springboard for nursing students, nursing educators, and practicing nurses. With a solid conceptual base and practical how-to ideas for family assessment and intervention, we hope that more nurses will gain confidence to engage in the nursing of families. In so doing, they will be reclaiming some aspects of nursing that have been given to other health professionals. In the process, nurses will regain an important dimension of nursing practice. We predict this will be quickly and readily appreciated by families requiring such care.

LMW
ML

ACKNOWLEDGMENTS

We are grateful to our colleagues, friends, families, and students for their nudging, support, and encouragement throughout the writing of this second edition.

In particular, we are grateful to:

Janice Bell, Fabie Duhamel, and Marilyn Friedman, who not only encouraged us but convinced us that a second edition had become a necessity.

Bob Martone and Ruth De George from F. A. Davis, who encouraged, prodded, and cheered us on to revise the first edition.

Crystal McNichol and Bob Butler from F. A. Davis, who helped transform our raw manuscript into this fine-tuned, finished product.

Janice Bell, Fabie Duhamel, Sandy Harper-Jaques, Sandra Hirst, Anne Marie Levac, Michele Nanchoff-Glatt, Loree Stout, and Wendy Watson, who so willingly reviewed and critiqued various chapters. These colleagues greatly enhanced the final outcome of this book.

Marlene Baier, who patiently assisted us in typing and retyping numerous drafts. We enjoyed her various comments in the margins.

LMW
ML

For each of us, there have been other individuals to whom we would like to express special thanks and appreciation:

I would like to express admiration and love to my dear friend and colleague, Wendy Watson, for 11 years of working together with nurses and families. Although this chapter of our professional lives has come to a close, our shared experiences of supervising nursing students, our own clinical work with families, and 1001 conversations about it all have contributed immeasurably to the ideas presented in this book.

LMW

I would like to thank my husband, and biggest fan, Douglas Leahey, for his unfailing interest in our progress on the second edition. His encouragement and compliments facilitated the completion of this work.

ML

Finally, we are grateful to each other. The first edition saw us progress from colleagues to friends. Ten years later, we continue to enjoy a very special mixing of friendship and collegueship through numerous telephone calls, meals, and trips. From Calgary to Czechoslovakia and from

Fort McMurray to Florida, we have co-constructed reality and enjoyed each other's company. We have also drawn ideas from our different work contexts, each a beautiful blend of education, practice, and research. The whole *is* greater than the sum of the parts, as is reflected in this book.

LMW
ML
February, 1994

CONTENTS

CHAPTER 1

FAMILY ASSESSMENT AND INTERVENTION: AN OVERVIEW

Nursing has come of age with its recognition of the significance of the family to the health and well-being of individual family members. Equally important, nursing has recognized the influence of the family on illness. The main evidence for these statements is in five areas: nursing practice, nursing education, nursing research of families, nursing literature, and family nursing conferences. Within each of these areas, new language has emerged to name, describe, and communicate this trend. Some new terms are "family-centered care" (Cunningham, 1978), "family-focused care" (Janosik & Miller, 1979), "family interviewing" (Wright & Leahey, 1984), "family health promotion nursing" (Bomar, 1989), "family nursing" (Bell, Watson, & Wright, 1990; Friedman, 1992; Gilliss, 1991; Gilliss, Highley, Roberts, & Martinson, 1989; Hanson, 1991; Leahey & Wright, 1987; McFarlane, 1986; Wegner & Alexander, 1993; Wright & Leahey, 1987a, 1987b; Wright & Leahey, 1990), "family systems nursing" (Wright & Leahey, 1990; Wright, Watson, & Bell, 1990), and "nursing of families" (Feetham, Meister, Bell, & Gilliss, 1993).

As nurses theorize about and involve families more in healthcare, they are altering or modifying their usual patterns of clinical practice. The implication for this change in practice is that nurses need to become competent in assessing and intervening with families. The required knowledge and clinical skills of these new competencies can be acquired most efficiently by studying the whole family unit rather than by studying each family member in isolation. By studying whole families, nurses will think about interaction and reciprocity. Specifically, the dominant focus of the competencies must be the reciprocity between health or illness and the family. It is most useful for nurses to assess the impact of illness on the family and the influence of family interaction on health or on the "cause," "course," or "cure" of illness. Another level of essential reciprocity in nursing practice is an assessment of the interaction between the patient/ family and the nurse. Health/illness, families, and nurses have each been studied as separate elements by a variety of disciplines. However, it is the study of the reciprocity or relationships *between* the elements that is new to nurses. Therefore, it is our belief that nursing of families must focus on relationships, not on discrete elements. To the present, there has been too much fascination, categorization, and research of these discrete elements. Systemic thinkers have been quick to see the fallacy of such a categorization (Wright & Bell, 1981). Fortunately, nursing is shifting toward a systemic understanding of families experiencing health problems.

EVOLUTION OF THE NURSING OF FAMILIES

In researching the beginnings of the nursing of families, we unearthed some interesting findings. One of the most significant of which is that involving families in healthcare has always been part of nursing but has not been labeled as such. Because nursing originated in patients' homes, it was natural to involve family members and to provide family-centered care. With the transition of nursing practice from homes to hospitals during the depression and World War II, families became excluded not only from involvement in caring for their ill member but from major family events such as birth and death. However, it now appears that with emphasis on inviting families "back" to participate in healthcare, nursing has come full circle. The history, evolution, and theory development of the nursing of families has recently been discussed in depth in the literature (Feetham, et al. 1993; Friedman, 1992; Gilliss, 1991; Gilliss, et al. 1989; Lansberry & Richards, 1992; Whall & Fawcett, 1991). These authors have made a significant contribution to the advancement of nursing knowledge by contextualizing nursing care with families. Nursing of families has come to mean nursing care of the well and the ill with emphasis on the responses of families to actual or potential health problems. Unfortunately, there is a gap between theory and ideals and actual clinical practice. Friedman (1992) contends that a "family-centered approach remains a stated ideal rather than a prevailing practice—not only in inpatient but also community and clinic settings" (p. xv). Laitinen's (1992) study confirms this, as he found that the participation of family members and relatives in patient hospital care is minimal.

We believe the most significant variable that promotes or impedes family-centered care is how a nurse conceptualizes problems. Sluzki (1974) suggests that the ability "to conceive [of] the individual as constantly defining and being defined by his relationships to his family and to other meaningful members of his milieu and by his insertion in the community at large" (p. 484) is perhaps more difficult for those who are already knowledgeable and well trained in an intrapersonal, psychological, or medical model than for beginning practitioners.

It is this ability to "think interactionally" that raises the delivery of healthcare from an individual to a family (interactional) level. Robinson (1992) offers a thought-provoking idea that "distinctions between individual and family nursing have been framed as dichotomies and so have become separations rather than simply perceptions of difference" (p. 2). She proposes conceptualizing nursing as inclusive of *both* individuals and families with distinctions made about the focus of practice. Robinson's (1992) ideas emerged from her application of Maturana's (1988) notion that not only are persons and families different kinds of systems but they also exist in different domains. Learning to make the transition from a more traditional individualistic perspective toward "thinking interactionally" or "thinking family" can be facilitated by providing nurses with a clear framework for assessing families and the necessary interventions to treat families.

FAMILY ASSESSMENT

There have been many attempts to define and conceptualize the family from multiple perspectives by numerous disciplines. Duvall (1977) lists a series of 15 of the social sciences and disciplines conducting research on one or more aspects of family life. These include anthropology, counseling, economics, human development, psychology, public health, religion, social work, and sociology. Each discipline has its own point of view or frame of reference for viewing the family. Economists, for example, have been concerned with how the family members work together to meet their material needs. Sociologists, on the other hand, are concerned with the family as a specific group in society. Nursing authors Liefson (1987) and Mischke-Berkey, Warner, and Hanson (1989) have identified and described several family assessment models and instruments developed by both nurses and others. This compilation of family assessment models and instruments is a very useful and worthwhile effort to make distinctions between models and the variables emphasized in each. There is no one assessment model, however, that explains *all* family phenomena.

In the clinical setting, it is useful for nurses to adopt a clear conceptual framework or a map of the family. This encourages the synthesis of data so that family strengths and problems can be identified and a useful management plan devised. When a conceptual framework is absent, it is extremely difficult for the nurse to group disparate data or examine the relationships among the multiple variables that have an impact on the family. The use of a family assessment framework helps to organize this massive amount of seemingly disparate information. It also provides a focus for intervention.

CALGARY FAMILY ASSESSMENT MODEL: AN INTEGRATED FRAMEWORK

The Calgary Family Assessment Model (CFAM) is a multidimensional framework consisting of three major categories: structural, developmental, and functional (Chapter 3). The model is based on a systems/cybernetics/communication/change theory foundation. It has been adapted from Tomm and Sanders's (1983) family assessment model and substantially embellished since our first edition of this book.

INDICATIONS AND CONTRAINDICATIONS FOR A FAMILY ASSESSMENT

It is important to identify some guidelines for determining *which* families will automatically be considered for family assessment. It is not a common practice in our society, as yet, to have families present themselves as a family unit for assistance with particular *family* problems. Rather, the problem is more frequently presented as isolated within a particular family member. Therefore, it is with each problem situation that a judgment must be made about whether that particular problem should be approached within a family context.

The following indications for a family assessment have been adapted from Clarkin, Frances, and Moodie (1979):

1. A family is experiencing emotional disruption caused by a family crisis (e.g., acute illness, injury, or death).
2. A family is experiencing emotional disruption caused by a developmental milestone (e.g., birth, marriage, or youngest child leaving home).
3. A family defines a problem as a family issue, and there is motivation for family assessment (e.g., the impact of chronic illness on the family).
4. A child or adolescent is the identified patient.
5. The family is experiencing issues that are serious enough to jeopardize family relationships (e.g., terminal illness or sexual or physical abuse).
6. A family member is about to be admitted to the hospital for psychiatric treatment.

We concur with Barker (1981) that the use of family assessment "does not absolve (the nurse) from assessing suicidal, homicidal and other risks in individual family members" (p. 86). Family assessment is neither a panacea nor a substitute for an individual assessment.

Some contraindications for family assessment are:

1. Individuation of a family member would be compromised by the family assessment. For example, if a young adult had recently left home for the first time, then a family interview may not be desirable.
2. Context of a family situation permits little or no leverage. That is, the family might have the fixed belief that the nurse is working as an agent of some other institution (e.g., the court).

During the engagement process, nurses need to be quite explicit in presenting the rationale for family assessment. Suggestions for how to do this are given in Chapters 6 and 7. In deciding whether to do a family assessment or not, the nurse should be guided by sound clinical principles and judgment. The nurse can take advantage of opportunities to consult with peers and supervisors should there be any questions about the suitability of such an assessment.

Once the nurse has completed the family assessment, she must decide if she will or will not intervene further with the family. In the next section of this chapter, we discuss our general ideas about intervention. Specific ideas for nurses to consider when making clinical decisions about interventions with particular families are presented in Chapters 4 and 7.

NURSING INTERVENTIONS: A GENERIC DISCUSSION

Numerous terms are used to distinguish and ultimately label the treatment portion of nursing practice: intervention, treatment, therapeutics, action, and activity (Bulechek & McCloskey, 1992b). In our clinical practice and research with families, we prefer the designation of *intervention.* The most rigorous efforts to contribute to a standardized language for nursing interventions is the work of Bulechek and McCloskey (1992a, 1992b) and their colleagues at the University of Iowa. We applaud their ambitious and much needed efforts to develop and validate nursing intervention labels. Because we perceive them as clearly providing leadership in this far-neglected area within nursing, we use their conceptualization and findings as our base of reference from which we agree and disagree.

First, however, we wish to present a brief overview of the evolutionary process of identifying, defining, and describing nursing interventions. In 1980, the American Nurses' Association (ANA) published *Nursing: A Social Policy Statement,* which stated that "nursing is the diagnosis and treatment of human responses to actual or potential health problems" (p. 9). Although ANA accepted the activity of nursing diagnoses, there continues to be much debate and controversy within the nursing profession about the nature and labels of nursing diagnoses (Bulechek & McCloskey, 1992a; Wright & Levac, 1992). At the ninth North American Nursing Diagnosis Association (NANDA) conference the following definition was accepted: "A nursing diagnosis is a clinical judgment about individual, family or community responses to actual or potential health problems/life processes. Nursing diagnoses provide the basis for selection of nursing interventions to achieve outcomes for which the nurse is accountable" (Carroll-Johnson, 1990, p. 50).

Bulechek and McCloskey (1992a) prefer to define a nursing diagnosis as "the identification of a patient's problem that the nurse can treat" (p. 5). This definition comes closest to expressing how we prefer to label the difficulties experienced by families; that is, following an assessment of a family, we prefer to generate a strengths and problems list rather than diagnoses. We conceptualize the strengths and problems list as one observer perspective, not the "truth" about a family. We view the problem list as problems that can be treated. It has been our experience that nursing diagnoses have unfortunately become too rigid. We agree with Bulechek and McCloskey (1992) that wellness diagnoses are not necessary, but for different reasons. We prefer to identify the strengths of the family and list them alongside their problems (Chapter 8). The advantage of this manner of classification is that it gives a balanced view of a family. It also invites us as nurses not to become blinded by a family's problems but to realize that every family has strengths even in the face of potential or actual health problems.

DEFINITION OF A NURSING INTERVENTION

Bulechek and McCloskey (1990) define a nursing intervention as "any direct care treatment that a nurse performs on behalf of a client which includes nurse-initiated treatments, physician-initiated treatments and performance of daily essential functions" (p. 26). Wright, Watson, and Bell (1993) offer an alternate definition: Any action or response of the nurse, which includes the nurse's overt therapeutic actions and internal cognitive/affect responses that occur in the context of a nurse-client relationship, to affect individual, family, or community functioning for which nurses are accountable.

CONTEXT OF A NURSING INTERVENTION

The focus of concern with a nursing intervention should be the nurse behavior *and* the family response. This differs from nursing diagnosis and nursing outcome, where the focus is client behavior (Bulechek & McCloskey, 1992). We believe nurse behaviors and client behaviors are contextualized in the nurse-client relationship. Therefore, an interactional phenomenon occurs whereby the responses of a nurse (interventions) are invited by the responses of clients (outcome), which in turn are invited by the responses of a nurse. To focus on only client behaviors *or* nurse behaviors does not take into account the relationship between nurses *and* clients. Haller (1990) makes an important point when she comments that interactional research is the study of relationships and states that "many of our nursing interventions are interactional; that is, not doing to or for the patient, but with the patient" (p. 272). We would submit that *all* nursing interventions are interactional. Nursing interventions are only actualized in a relationship.

INTENT OF NURSING INTERVENTIONS

The intent of any nursing intervention is to effect change. Therefore, effective nursing interventions (i.e., particular perturbations) are those that clients/families respond to because of the fit between the intervention offered by the nurse and the psychobiological structure of the client (Wright & Levac, 1992).

NURSING INTERVENTIONS WITH FAMILIES: A SPECIFIC DISCUSSION

There are numerous ways in which to intervene with families. This section discusses some specific aspects of interventions with families. It also presents indications and contraindications for family intervention.

CONCEPTUALIZATION OF INTERVENTIONS WITH FAMILIES

Keeney (1982) has defined interventions with families as the introduction of new pieces of information into family systems that may help families to behave differently. With regard to interventions, it is unwise to attempt to ascertain what is "really" going on with a particular family or what the "real" problem is; what is real to us as nurses, whether it be the problem or the intervention, is always a consequence of our social construction of the world (Keeney, 1982). Keeney further states that because family clinicians join their clients in the social construction of a therapeutic reality, the clinician is also responsible "for the universe of experience that is created" (p. 165). Maturana (1988) presents another aspect of this critical notion of reality by submitting that individuals (living systems) draw forth reality—they do not construct it and it does not exist independent of them. This has implications for nurses' clinical work with families in that what we perceive about particular situations with families is obtained by how we behave (our interventions), and how we behave depends on what we perceive.

Therefore, one way to change the reality that family members have drawn forth is to assist them in the development of new ways of interacting in the family. The interventions we use in this endeavor are focused on changing cognitive, affective, or behavioral domains of family functioning. As family members' perceptions about each other and the illness change, so will their behavior. Thus interventions normally are directed at challenging the meanings or beliefs that families give to behavioral events (Watson, Bell, & Wright, 1992; Watson & Nanchoff-Glatt, 1990; Wright, Bell, & Rock, 1989; Wright & Nagy, 1993; Wright & Simpson, 1991; Wright & Watson, 1988).

We must also keep in mind the element of time with regard to interventions. Interventions do not just begin with the intervention stage of family work. Rather, they are an integral part of family interviewing, spanning engagement to termination. Normally, interventions used during the specific intervention stage of family interviewing are based on the nurse's assessment of the family. If there has been adequate engagement and assessment of the family, then this will generally increase the effectiveness of the interventions. For example, if in working with a Latino family, the nurse perpetually addresses family members other than the father first, the family may disengage. The opportunity to intervene further will be eliminated. In this example, one needs not only to possess family interviewing skills but also sensitivity to ethnic issues before embarking on specific goal-oriented interventions.

INDICATIONS AND CONTRAINDICATIONS FOR FAMILY INTERVENTIONS

Following a family assessment, nurses have to decide whether or not to intervene with a family. They need to consider the family's level of functioning, their own skill level, and the resources available. We have drawn up some indicators for family intervention beyond the initial interviews (Leahey and Wright, 1987) and have recommended intervention under the following circumstances (pp. 66–67):

- A family member presents with an . . . illness that has an obvious detrimental impact on the other family members. For instance, a grandfather's Alzheimer's disease may result in the grandchildren being afraid of him or a young child's acting out behavior may be related to his mother's deterioration from multiple sclerosis.
- Family members contribute to an individual's symptoms or problems as when lack of visitation from adult children exacerbates hypochondriasis in an elderly parent.
- One member's improvement leads to symptoms or deterioration in another family member, for example, when decreased asthma symptoms in one child correlate with increased abdominal pain in a sibling.
- A child or adolescent develops an emotional, behavioral, or physical problem in the context of a family member's . . . illness. Perhaps a diabetic adolescent suddenly requests that his mother give him his daily insulin injections when he has been injecting himself for the past 6 months.
- A family member is first diagnosed with an . . . illness. If a family has no previous knowledge or experience with a particular illness, it will require information.
- A family member's condition deteriorates markedly. Whenever there is deterioration, family patterns will need restructuring, and intervention is indicated.
- A chronically ill family member moves from a hospital or rehabilitation center back into the community.
- An important individual or family developmental milestone is missed or delayed, such as when an adolescent is unable to move out of the home at the anticipated time.
- The chronically ill patient dies. Even though the patient's death may be a relief, the family can be faced with a tremendous void where the caretaking role used to be.

After the nurse has decided that intervention is indicated, the nurse and family must then decide on the duration and intensity of the family sessions. If sessions occur too frequently, there may be insufficient delay time for the family's feedback mechanisms to process the change. The optimal exact number of days, weeks, or months between sessions is difficult to state categorically. We recommend that nurses ask the family members when they would like to have another meeting. In our clinical experience, families are much better judges than nurses of how frequently they need to be seen to resolve a particular problem. Furthermore, nurses should be aware that the duration and intensity of sessions depends on the context in which the family is seen. For example, if a hospital nurse is working with a family, the nurse and family would perhaps schedule a few sessions in the early part of the patient's hospitalization and then decrease the number of sessions prior to the patient's being discharged. In this way, the family would have the opportunity to gradually terminate with the hospital staff. Additional information on termination is discussed in Chapter 9.

Given that family intervention is not always required, the question arises about the *contraindications* for family intervention. These include:

1. *All* family members state that they do not wish to pursue family treatment even though it is recommended.
2. The family states that they agree with the recommendation for family treatment but would prefer to work with another professional.

These contraindications are generally evident to the nurse immediately following the family assessment. Sometimes during the course of intervention, however, families indicate a desire to terminate treatment. We discuss this situation more fully in Chapter 9.

It is evident that nurses working with patients and families in a variety of healthcare settings need to have a good understanding of when family involvement is indicated and when it is contraindicated. Not only for their own benefit but also for the family's benefit, nurses should make a distinction between family assessment and family intervention. Families often are willing to come for an assessment where they can see the nurse face to face and make *their* own assessment of the interviewer's competency. If a nurse does a careful, credible assessment, then she will have an easier time in doing family intervention work.

DEVELOPMENT AND IDENTIFICATION OF NURSING INTERVENTIONS WITH FAMILIES

Craft and Willadsen (1992) state that "the development of nursing interventions with families has been hampered by the lack of nursing theory of family" (p. 517). They further suggest that the specification, validation, and testing of interventions related to family is relatively novel for nursing. We concur with these thoughts but also believe that the lack of specific interventions with families has been due to the lack of nurse educators who are skilled family clinicians. Because interventions related to family are independent nursing interventions for which nurses are accountable (Wright, Watson, & Bell, 1993), nurse educators and researchers must begin specifying and testing interventions related to family (Craft & Willadsen, 1992). It is not surprising that there have been very few tested nursing interventions with families when our profession is at a very neophyte stage of even identifying and describing family interventions.

The recent efforts by Craft and Willadsen (1992) are a major contribution to assisting nursing practice to specify and validate family interventions and eventually to test them. They conducted a study that surveyed 130 nurse experts in the United States, of whom 54 (41 percent) responded. From their findings, Craft and Willadsen (1992) conclude that "nursing intervention levels related to family can be specified in a manner that has common meaning to experts in family nursing" (p. 524). Specifically, this study labeled, defined, and gave critical and supporting activities for nine interventions related to family: family support, family process maintenance, family integrity promotion, family involvement, family mobilization, caregiver support, sibling support, parent education, and family therapy.

Craft and Willadsen's (1992) study is an important beginning. Efforts now need to be made to validate these identified interventions through both clinical and empirical means (Feetham, 1992). We suggest that it would be useful in future studies attempting to label family interventions to specify the amount of clinical contact the experts have with families. We believe nurses in direct clinical contact with families perceive family interventions differently than nurses who predominantly conduct research or engage in theory development. We found Craft and Willadsen's labeling, defining, and citing of specific activities of nine interventions to be useful, but we believe that some of the descriptions of critical and supporting activities for each intervention may be more congruent with family assessment than with intervention (e.g., "determine how patient behavior affects family; identify family member's perceptions of the situations and precipitating events"). We do agree with their identification and descriptions of all but one of the interventions cited—we disagree with the labeling of family therapy as an intervention. We believe this to be a conceptual error.

Family therapy is *not* an intervention. Family therapy is much more than an intervention. "It is a world view that involves a conceptual shift from linear to systems (systemic) thinking" (Watson, 1992, p. 379). Family therapy is not only a particular type of clinical practice with families but is also a distinct profession. Since 1978, the American Association for Marriage and Family Therapy's Commission on Accreditation has been recognized by the United States Department of Education as the professional body that defines the practice and the profession of family therapy. At the same time, specialization in family therapy can and does occur within nursing, social work, psychology, and psychiatry.

"Non-family therapists often view family therapy as: a) a modality, that b) usually involves a nuclear family. Family therapy is *not* simply a 'modality.' Nor is it necessarily a set of modalities. More fundamentally, it is a way of construing human problems that dictates certain actions for their alleviation" (Stanton, 1988, pp. 7–8). We strongly concur with Watson (1992) and Stanton (1988) and submit that the "actions" that Stanton refers to are interventions. This does not mean that nurses cannot be educated and trained in the practice of family therapy, but that it must be provided at the graduate (master or doctoral) or postgraduate (post-baccalaureate) level. Family therapy specialization within nursing can be coherent if there is more openness within both disciplines and if one does not attempt to consume the other (Wright & Leahey, 1988).

The education and training of students in clinical work with families at the undergraduate level primarily focuses on the family as context (Wright & Leahey, 1990). Nursing students specializing in family systems nursing (Wright & Leahey, 1990; Wright, Watson, & Bell, 1990) are at the graduate or advanced practice level (Calkin, 1984). Thus it is extremely important that our efforts to label interventions be consistent within a particular practice framework: interventions with family as context, interventions within family systems nursing, or interventions within family therapy. However, it is possible that some interventions labeled within one domain of clinical practice with families may be identifiable in another domain of clinical practice.

NURSING PRACTICE LEVELS WITH FAMILIES: GENERALIST AND SPECIALIST

Lansberry and Richards (1992) emphasize that nursing practice with families is directed by whether the family is conceptualized as "family as context" or "family as client." They believe that a different belief system informs each type of practice with families. Specifically, the totality paradigm beliefs inform family as context, and the simultaneity paradigm beliefs inform family as client (Lansberry & Richards, 1992). One way to alleviate any potential confusion of practice levels is to make a clear distinction between two levels of *expertise* in nursing with regard to clinical work with families: generalists and specialists (Wright & Leahey, 1988). Typically, generalists are nurses at the baccalaureate level who are predominantly using the conceptualization of the family as context (Wright & Leahey, 1990). Specialists, on the other hand, are nurses who are at the graduate (master or doctoral) level who are predominantly using the conceptualization of the family as the unit or client of care. This requires specialization in "family systems nursing" (Wright & Leahey, 1990). Family systems nursing specialization requires that "the focus is always on interaction and reciprocity. It is not 'either/or' but rather 'both/and'. Family systems nursing is the integration of nursing, systems, cybernetics and family therapy theories" (Wright and Leahey, 1990, p. 149). It requires familiarity with an extensive body of knowledge: family dynamics, family systems theory, family assessment, family intervention, and family research. It also requires accompanying competence in family interviewing skills. Family systems nursing focuses on *both* the family system and individual systems simultaneously (Wright & Leahey, 1990).

We no longer subscribe to the term *family nursing* of which we once wrote (Wright & Leahey, 1990) because we no longer believe that family nursing is an appropriate term to define a baccalaureate nurse's involvement with families. We do believe that this term has served a useful purpose within our profession, as it sensitized nurses to reinvolve families in healthcare. We now prefer the term *nursing of families,* as it captures an aspect of nursing at the generalist level. All nurses should be knowledgeable and competent about the nursing of families, just as it is expected that they should be knowledgeable about nursing ethics or pharmacology, which also cut across all domains of nursing practice. Consequently, the emphasis in the practice of nursing of families at the generalist level is the family as context.

In contrast, the practice of family systems nursing at the specialist level emphasizes the family as the unit of care. However, we do admit that these boundaries may and can become blurred with upper-level baccalaureate students, who recognize the important focus on reciprocity and deal with individual and family systems simultaneously.

CONCLUSIONS

We consider it a great privilege to work with families experiencing health problems. We are also grateful for opportunities to teach professional nurses and nursing students about how to involve families in healthcare. Through this process, we recognize the extreme importance of nurses' having sound family assessment and intervention knowledge and skills. The remainder of this book is our effort to assist nurses to assist families.

REFERENCES

Barker, P. (1981). *Basic family therapy.* Baltimore: University Park Press.

Bell, J. M., Watson, W. L., & Wright, L. M. (Eds.). (1990). *The cutting edge of family nursing.* Calgary, Alberta: Family Nursing Unit Publications.

Bomar, P. J. (Ed.). (1989). *Nurses and family health promotion: Concepts, assessment and interventions.* Baltimore: Williams & Wilkins.

Bulechek, G. M., & McCloskey, J. C. (1990). Nursing interventions: Taxonomy development. In J. C. McCloskey & H. K. Grace (Eds.), *Current issues in nursing* (3rd ed., pp. 23–28), St. Louis: C. V. Mosby.

Bulechek, G. M., & McCloskey, J. C. (Eds.). (1992a). Defining and validating nursing interventions. *Nursing Clinics of North America, 27*(2), 289–297.

Bulechek, G. M., & McCloskey, J. C. (Eds.). (1992b). *Nursing interventions: Essential nursing treatments.* Philadelphia: W. B. Saunders.

Calkin, J. C. (1984) A model for advanced nursing practice. *Journal of Nursing Administration, 14*(1), 24–30.

Carroll-Johnson, R. M. (1990). Reflections on the ninth biennial conferences. *Nursing Diagnosis, 1,* 50.

Clarkin, J., Frances, A., & Moodie, J. (1979). Selection criteria for family therapy. *Family Process, 18,* 391–404.

Cousins, N. (1979). *Anatomy of an illness as perceived by the patient.* New York: Bantam Books.

Craft, M. J., & Willadsen, J. A. (1992). Interventions related to family. *Nursing Clinics of North America, 27*(2), 517–540.

Cunningham, R. (1978). Family-centered care. *Canadian Nurse, 2,* 34–37.

Doherty, W. J. (1985). Family interventions in health care. *Family Relations. 34,* 129–137.

Duvall, E. (1977). *Marriage and family development* (5th ed.). New York: Harper & Row.

Feetham, S. (1992). Family outcomes: Conceptual and methodological issues. In P. Moritz (Ed.), *Proceedings of patient outcomes research: Examining the effectiveness of nursing practice* (pp. 103–111). Bethesda, MD: National Center for Nursing Research, National Institutes of Health.

Feetham, S. L., Meister, S. B., Bell, J. M., & Gilliss, C. L. (1993). *The nursing of families: Theory, research, education and practice.* Newbury Park, CA: Sage.

Friedman, M. M. (1992). *Family nursing: Theory and practice.* East Norwalk, CT: Appleton & Lange.

Gilliss, C. L. (1991). Family nursing research, theory and practice. *Image: Journal of Nursing Scholarship,* 23(1), 19–22.

Gilliss, C. L., Highley, B. L., Roberts, B. M., & Martinson, I. M. (Eds.). (1989). *Toward a science of family nursing.* Menlo Park, CA: Addison-Wesley.

Haller, K. B. (1990). Characteristics of interactional research. *MCN, 15,* 272.

Hanson, S. (1991). Pocket guide to family assessment and intervention. St. Louis: C. V. Mosby.

Janosik, E., & Miller, J. (1979). Theories of family development. In D. Hymovich & M. Barnard (Eds.), *Family health care: Vol. 1. General perspectives* (2nd ed., pp. 3–16). New York: McGraw-Hill.

Keeney, B. (1982). What is an epistemology of family therapy? *Family Process, 21,* 153–168.

Laitinen, P. (1992). Participation of informal caregivers in the hospital care of elderly patients and their evaluation of the care giver: Pilot study in three different hospitals. *Journal of Advanced Nursing, 17,* 1233–1237.

Lansberry, C. R., & Richards, E. (1992). Family nursing practice paradigm perspectives and diagnostic approaches. *Advances in Nursing Science, 15*(2), 66–75.

Leahey, M., & Wright, L. M. (1987). Families and chronic illness: Assumptions, assessment and intervention. In L. M. Wright & M. Leahey (Eds.), *Families & chronic illness* (pp. 55–76). Springhouse, PA: Springhouse.

Leifson, J. (1987). Assessing families of infants with congenital defects. In L. M. Wright & M. Leahey (Eds.), *Families and chronic illness.* Springhouse, PA: Springhouse.

Maturana, H. (1988). Reality: The search for objectivity or the quest for a compelling argument. *Irish Journal of Psychology, 6*(1): 25–83.

McFarlane, J. M. (1986). *The clinical handbook of family nursing.* New York: John Wiley & Sons.

Mischke-Berkey, K., Warner, P., & Hanson, S. (1989). Family health assessment and intervention. In P. J. Bomar (Ed.), *Nurses and family health promotion: Concepts, assessment, and interventions* (pp. 115–154). Baltimore: Williams & Wilkins.

Robinson, C. (1992). *Beyond dichotomies in the nursing of persons and families.* Unpublished manuscript.

Sluzki, C. (1974). On training to think interactionally. *Social Science and Medicine, 8,* b483–485.

Stanton, D. M. (1988). The lobster quadrille: Issues and dilemmas for family therapy research. In L. C. Wynne (Ed.), *The state of the art in family therapy research: Controversies and recommendations* (pp. 5–31). New York: Family Process Press.

Tomm, K., & Sanders, G. (1983). Family assessment in a problem oriented record. In J. C. Hansen & B. F. Keeney (Eds.), *Diagnosis and assessment in family therapy* (pp. 101–122). London: Aspen Systems.

Watson, W. L. (1992). Family therapy. In G. M. Bulechek & J. C. McCloskey (Eds.), *Nursing interventions: Essential nursing treatments* (pp. 379–391). Philadelphia: W. B. Saunders.

Watson, W. L., Bell, J. M., & Wright, L. M. (1992). Osteophytes and marital fights: A single case clinical research report of chronic pain. *Family Systems Medicine, 10*(4), 423–435.

Watson, W. L., & Nanchoff-Glatt, M. (1990). A family systems nursing approach to premenstrual syndrome. *Clinical Nurse Specialist, 4,* 3–9.

Wegner, G. D., & Alexander, R. J. (Eds.). (1993). *Readings in family nursing.* Philadelphia: J. B. Lippincott.

Whall, A. L., & Fawcett, J. (Eds.). (1991). *Family theory development in nursing: State of the science and art.* Philadelphia: F. A. Davis.

Wright, L. M., & Bell, J. (1981). Nurses, families, and illness: A new combination. In D. Freeman & B. Trute (Eds.), *Treating families with special needs* (pp. 199–205). Ottawa, Ontario: Canadian Association of Social Workers.

Wright, L. M., Bell, J. M., & Rock, B. L. (1989). Smoking behavior and spouses: A case report. *Family Systems Medicine, 7*(2), 158–171.

Wright, L. M., & Leahey, M. (1984). *Nurses and families. A guide to family assessment and intervention.* Philadelphia: F. A. Davis.

Wright, L. M., & Leahey, M. (1987a). Families and life-threatening illness: Assumptions, assessment and intervention. In M. Leahey & L. M. Wright (Eds.), *Families & life-threatening illness* (pp. 45–58). Springhouse, PA: Springhouse.

Wright, L. M., & Leahey, M. (1987b). Families and pyschosocial problems: Assumptions, assessment and intervention. In M. Leahey & L. M. Wright (Eds.), *Families & psychosocial problems* (pp. 17–34). Springhouse, PA: Springhouse.

Wright, L. M., & Leahey, M. (1988). Nursing and family therapy training. In H. A. Liddle, D. C. Breunlin, & R. C. Schwartz (Eds.), *Handbook of family therapy training and supervision* (pp. 278–289). New York: Guilford Press.

Wright, L. M., & Leahey, M. (1990). Trends in the nursing of families. *Journal of Advanced Nursing, 15,* 148–154.

Wright, L. M., & Levac, A. M. (1992). The non-existence of non-compliant families: The influence of Humberto Maturana. *Journal of Advanced Nursing, 17,* 913–917.

Wright, L. M., & Nagy, J. (1993). Death: The most troublesome family secret of all. In E. Imber-Black (Ed.), *Secrets in families and family therapy* (pp. 121–137). New York: W. W. Norton.

Wright, L. M., & Simpson, P. (1991). A systemic belief approach to epileptic seizures: A case of being spellbound. *Contemporary Family Therapy: An International Journal, 13*(2), 165–180.

Wright, L. M., & Watson, W. L. (1988). Systemic family therapy and family development. In C. J. Falicov (Ed.), *Family transitions: Continuity and change over the life cycle* (pp. 407–430). New York: Guilford Press.

Wright, L. M., Watson, W. L., & Bell, J. M. (1990). The Family Nursing Unit: A unique integration of research, education and clinical practice. In J. M. Bell, W. L. Watson, & L. M. Wright (Eds.), *The cutting edge of family nursing* (pp. 95–109). Calgary, Alberta: Family Nursing Unit Publications.

Wright, L. M., Watson, W. L., & Bell, J. M. (1993). Personal communication.

2

THEORETICAL FOUNDATIONS OF THE CALGARY FAMILY ASSESSMENT AND INTERVENTION MODELS

To comprehend and use the Calgary Family Assessment Model (Chapter 3) and the Calgary Family Intervention Model (Chapter 4) in nursing practice with families, it is important to know the theoretical assumptions underlying these models. The underlying theoretical assumptions of family assessment and intervention models are important to declare for they are the foundation of how those models are operationalized. The four theoretical foundations that inform the models and practice presented in the rest of this textbook are: systems theory, cybernetics, communication theory, and change theory. Each theory, with some of the distinguishing concepts, is presented and related to families.

SYSTEMS THEORY

General systems theory, introduced in 1936 by von Bertalanffy, has been applied with increasing frequency by health professionals to the study of families. In addition to the original writings on systems theory by von Bertalanffy (1968, 1972, 1974), numerous articles and chapters in books have been written on systems theory and its concepts. This proliferation of systems information is also evident within nursing literature.

One of the most useful analogies that highlights systems concepts as applied to families is offered by Allmond, Buckman, and Gofman (1979).

They suggest that when thinking of a family as a system it is useful to compare it to a mobile.

> Visualize a mobile with four or five pieces suspended from the ceiling, gently moving in the air. The whole is in balance, steady yet moving. Some pieces are moving rapidly; others are almost stationary. Some are heavier and appear to carry more weight in the ultimate direction of the mobile's movement; others seem to go along for the ride. A breeze catching only one segment of the mobile immediately influences movement of every piece, some more than others, and the pace picks up with some pieces unbalancing themselves and moving chaotically about for a time. Gradually the whole exerts its influence in the errant part(s) and balance is reestablished but not before a decided change in direction of the whole may have taken place. You will also notice the changeability regarding closeness and distance among pieces, the impact of actual contact one with another, and the importance of vertical hierarchy. Coalitions of movement may be observed between two pieces. Or one piece may persistently appear isolated from the others; yet its position of isolation is essential to the balancing of the entire system. (p. 16)

Keeping the analogy of the mobile in mind, some of the most useful concepts of systems theory, which have frequent application in clinical practice with families, are highlighted below. These systems concepts provide a theoretical foundation for understanding the family as a system. A system can be defined as a complex of elements in mutual interaction. When this definition is applied to families, it allows us to view the family as a unit and thus focus on observing the interaction among family members rather than studying family members individually. However, it is to be remembered that each individual family member is both a subsystem and a system. An individual system is *both* a part and a whole as is a family.

Concept 1: A family system is part of a larger suprasystem and is also composed of many subsystems.

The concept of hierarchy of systems is very useful when applied to families. A family is composed of many subsystems such as parent-child, marital, and sibling subsystems. These subsystems are also composed of subsystems of individuals. Individuals are very complex systems composed of various subsystems, be they physical (e.g., cardiovascular, reproductive), or psychological (e.g., cognitive, affective). The family is also, at the same time, one unit nested in larger suprasystems such as neighborhoods, organizations, or church communities. Chin (1977) suggests that it is helpful to visualize a system by drawing a large circle and placing the elements, parts, or variables inside the circle. Then inside the circle, lines can be drawn among the component parts, which could be thought of as rubber bands or springs that stretch or contract as the forces increase or decrease. Outside of the circle is the larger context where all other factors impinging on the system may be placed. Thus a nurse can draw a circle to visualize a family and then place the individual family members within it (Fig. 2–1).

Systems are arbitrarily defined by their boundaries. Boundaries aid in specifying what is inside or outside the system. Normally, boundaries are associated with living systems of a physical nature, such as the number of people in a family or the skin of an individual. It is also possible to construct a boundary and, therefore, to create a system around ideas, beliefs, expectations, or roles. For example, there could be a system of multiple roles of a person or religious beliefs.

When working with families it is most useful to initially consider (1) who is in *this* family system, (2) what are some of the important subsystems, and (3) what are some of the significant suprasystems to which the family belongs. From time to time, however, it may be useful to draw a boundary (in one's mind) and create a system of beliefs, for example, parental beliefs about the use of corporal punishment with children.

Also, within family systems and their subsystems it is useful to assess the amount of permeability of the boundaries. In family systems, the boundary must be both permeable and limiting. If the family boundary is too permeable, the system loses its identity and integrity (e.g., too open to

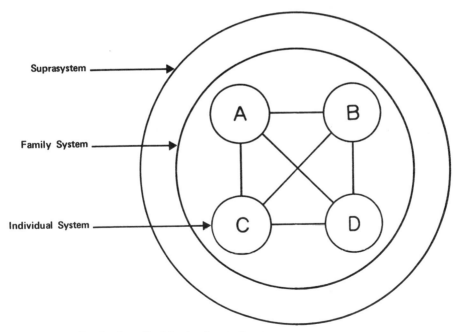

Figure 2–1. The family as it relates to other systems.

ideas and input from the outside environment) and therefore does not allow the family to use its own resources in decision making. However, if it is too closed or impermeable, the necessary input or interaction with the larger world is shut off (e.g., an immigrant family from Vietnam that relocates to Iowa may inadvertently remain closed initially due to great differences in language and culture largely defined by the information or communication that crosses over) (Barker, 1981).

The concept of hierarchy of systems and the boundaries that create systems is a most useful concept to apply when working with and attempting to conceptualize the uniqueness of each particular family.

Concept 2: The family as a whole is greater than the sum of its parts.

This concept of systems theory applied to families emphasizes that the family's "wholeness" is more than simply the addition of each family member. It also emphasizes that individuals are best understood within their larger context, which normally is the family. To study individual family members separately is not the same as studying the family as a unit. By studying the whole family, it is possible to observe the interaction among family members, which often explains more fully individual family member functioning. For example, a young mother complains to the Community Health Nurse (CHN) that her 3-year-old child has temper tantrums that she is not able to control, and asks for guidance. The CHN could intervene in a variety of ways: (1) see the mother individually and discuss some behavioral methods that could be used to assist in controlling her child's temper tantrums, (2) see the child individually and do an individual assessment, or (3) see the whole family (mother, father, and child) and do a child and family assessment (Chapter 3) in order to understand the child, the child's behavior in the family context, and the family.

The CHN chose to see the whole family because she understood the importance of concept 2. During the first session with the family, the child was very well behaved in the interview for the first quarter hour. Then the child had a temper tantrum, as a result of which the mother became annoyed and the father withdrew. The CHN was astute enough to observe the sequence of interaction prior to the temper tantrum. Right before the child had the temper tantrum, the parents were in a heated argument about their parenting styles. When the child had the temper tantrum, the parents stopped arguing and focused on the child. This child most likely was responding to the tension between the parents and thus the temper tantrums invited the parents to stop their conflict. The temper tantrums were consequently understood quite differently in the context of the family than they would have been if the child had been assessed in isolation.

Therefore, it is important that nurses see *whole* families when possible, to more fully understand family member functioning by observing family interaction. This enables an appreciation of the relationships that exist among family members as well as individual family member functioning. Ranson (1984) emphasizes this point by stating that "we cannot understand the parts of a body, a family, a practice, a theory, unless we know how the whole works, for the parts can be understood only in relation to the whole; conversely, we cannot grasp how the whole works unless we have an understanding of its parts" (p. 231).

> **Concept 3:** A change in one family member affects all family members.

This concept assists in the recognition that any significant event or change in one family member will affect all family members in varying degrees as illustrated in the analogy of the mobile. The concept can be most useful to nurses when thinking of the impact of illness on the family. For example, the father of a family experienced a coronary, the impact of which affected all family members and various family member relationships. The father and mother were unable to continue their active interest in sports together and the mother increased her employment from part-time to full-time in order to supplement their substantially reduced income during the father's convalescence. The eldest daughter, who had been more remote from the family since her marriage, began visiting her father more. The youngest daughter, by providing emotional support, became closer to her mother. Thus all family members were affected, and the usual organization and functioning of the family were changed.

This concept can also be applied to understand the impact of intervening in a family system. That is, if one family member begins to change, other family members will be unable to respond as they have previously because one family member is now behaving differently.

> **Concept 4:** The family is able to create a balance between change and stability.

Recently, there has been a shift in nursing away from the belief that families tend toward maintaining equilibrium and toward the belief that families are really in a constant state of flux. Thus the pendulum has swung from one end of the continuum to the other, from conceptualizing families as always maintaining equilibrium to always changing. However, von Bertalanffy (1968) warned us some years ago to avoid this polarized view of families. He suggested that systems, and in this case family systems, are able to achieve a balance among the forces operating in them and on them and that change and stability can coexist in living systems (see Change Theory in this chapter).

However, when change occurs in a family, there is a shift to a new position of balance after the disturbance. The family reorganizes in a way that is different from any previous organization of the family. For example, if a family member has been diagnosed with multiple sclerosis, the entire family will have to reorganize itself in ways that are totally different from before the diagnosis. The balance between change and stability will constantly shift in periods of remission and exacerbation, but more often there will be a balance between change and stability.

The concept of change and stability coexisting is perhaps one of the most difficult concepts of systems theory for nurse family interviewers to understand. This is due in part to the fact that in actual clinical practice, families will frequently present themselves "as if" they are in total equilibrium, *or* "as if" they are constantly changing, rather than manifesting an observable balance between the two. However, the more experienced one becomes in family work, the greater appreciation one has for the complexity of families. When families are "stuck" or experiencing severe difficulties, it is frequently because they are polarized in maintaining rigid equilibrium or are in a phase of too much change. Eventually, the family will need to find solutions to obtain a balance between the phenomena of stability and change.

> **Concept 5:** Family members' behaviors are best understood from a view of circular rather than linear causality.

One method of dealing with the massive amounts of data presented in a family interview is to observe for patterns. Tomm (1981) offers a very useful discussion of the differences between linear and circular patterns.

> One major difference between linear and circular patterns lies in the overall structure of the connections between elements of the pattern. Linear patterns are limited to sequences (e.g., A → B → C) whereas circular patterns form a closed loop and are recursive (e.g., A → B → C → A → ... or A → B, B → C, C → A). A less obvious but more significant difference lies in the relative importance usually given to *time* and *meaning* when making the connections or links in the pattern. Linearity is heavily rooted in a framework of a continuous progression of time . . . *Circularity* . . . is more heavily dependent on *a framework of reciprocal relationships based on meaning.* (p. 85)

Linear causality, defined as one event causing another, can serve a useful and helpful function for individuals and families. For example, when the clock strikes 6:00 PM, a family will routinely eat supper. This is an example of linear causality because event A (the clock striking 6:00 PM) is seen as the cause of event B (the eating of supper) (A → B), whereas event B does not affect event A (Barker, 1981).

However, circular causality occurs when event B *does* affect event A. For example, if a spouse takes an interest in his wife's ostomy care (event A) and the wife responds by explaining the daily procedures (event B), then it is likely to result in the husband continuing to take an interest and offer support regarding his wife's ostomy care and his wife feeling supported; thus the cycle continues (A → B → A). Each individual's behavior has an effect on and influences the other. A method for diagramming these circular patterns will be discussed in Chapter 3.

The application of these concepts in clinical practice affects the interviewer's style of questioning during a family interview. Linear questions tend to explore *descriptive* characteristics (e.g., "Is the father fearful of another heart attack?"), whereas circular questions tend to explore *differences* (e.g., "Who's the most worried about the father having another heart attack?") (Selvini-Palazzoli, Boscolo, Cecchin, & Prata, 1980; Tomm, 1984). Bateson (1979) offers the idea that "information consists of differences that make a difference" (p. 99).

> Differences between perceptions/objects/events/ideas/etc. are regarded as the basic source of all information and consequent knowledge. On closer examination, one can see that such *relationships are always reciprocal or circular.* If she is shorter than he, then he is taller than she. If she is dominant, then he is submissive. If one member of the family is defined as being bad, then the others are being defined as being good. Even at a very simple level, a circular orientation allows implicit information to become more explicit and offers alternative points of view. A linear orientation on the other hand is narrow and restrictive and tends to mask important data. (Tomm, 1981, p. 93)

Various types of assessment and interventive questions that could be asked during a family interview are highlighted in Chapters 3, 4, 6, and 7.

With regard to family member interaction, the assumption is made that each person mutually contributes to adaptive as well as maladaptive interaction. For example, a common problem presented in geriatric healthcare facilities is that the elderly parent complains that the adult children do not visit enough and, therefore, frequently withdraws while the adult children complain that their elderly parent constantly nags them when visiting. Each is "correct" in the perception of the other but does not recognize how each person's behavior influences the behavior of the other.

Normally, families and individual family members need to be assisted to move from a linear perspective of their situation to a systemic one. This is only possible if the nurse does not become caught in linear thinking when attempting to understand family dynamics.

These five concepts are by no means inclusive of all systems concepts but reflect those deemed the most significant and important to serve as a theoretical foundation when working with families.

CYBERNETICS

Cybernetics is the science of communication and control theory. The term was originally coined by a mathematician, Norbert Weiner. Beer (1974) indicated that "for some, cybernetics and General Systems Theory are co-extensive, while those could be found who regard each as a branch of the other" (p. 2). We believe it is important that general systems theory be differentiated from cybernetics and we do not use these terms synonymously. General systems theory is primarily concerned with changing our conceptual lens from parts to wholes, whereas cybernetics changes our focus from substance to form (Keeney, 1982). In the study of cybernetics, "both parts and wholes are examined in terms of their patterns of organization" (Keeney, 1982, p. 155).

> **Concept 1:** Families possess self-regulating ability through the process of feedback.

Interpersonal systems, particularly families, "may be viewed as feedback loops, since the behavior of each person affects and is affected by the behavior of each other person" (Watzlawick, Beavin, & Jackson, 1967, p. 31). For any substantial change to occur in a relationship, the regulatory limits must be adjusted so that a new range of behaviors is possible or an entirely new pattern can emerge (transformation) (Tomm, 1980, p. 8). Tomm (1980) has offered a useful method of applying cybernetic regulatory concepts in actual clinical interviewing. His method of diagramming circular patterns of communication will be discussed in Chapter 3.

> **Concept 2:** Feedback processes can simultaneously occur at several different systems levels with families.

Initially, the application of cybernetic concepts in family work began by observations of simple phenomena (e.g., wife criticizes, husband withholds), generally referred to as simple cybernetics. However, as cyberneticians began examining more complex orders of phenomena, there developed a recognition of different orders of feedback (e.g., feedback of feedback, change of change). "Margaret Mead suggested that the field call this perspective of higher-order process 'cybernetics of cybernetics' " (Keeney, 1982, p. 158). Maturana and Varela (1980) suggest a higher-order cybernetics that links the organization of living process and cognition. A further labeling by von Foerester (1974) makes the distinction between first-order cybernetics, or the cybernetics of simple feedback, and second-order cybernetics, or the cybernetics of cybernetics.

Therefore, the simple feedback phenomenon observed in the interactional pattern of criticizing wife–withholding husband may also be understood to be part of a larger feedback loop involving the couple's relationship to their families of origin, which may recalibrate the lower-order loop of the couple's interaction. Thus, cybernetics of cybernetics moves into a larger context, which includes both the observer and the observed. There is a recursive analysis that emphasizes the internal structure of the system and the mutual connectedness of the observer and the observed (Varela, 1979). Keeney (1983) suggests that the "cybernetic system we discern is a consequence of the distinctions we happen to draw" (p. 142).

COMMUNICATION THEORY

The focus of the study of communication is how individuals interact with one another. One of the most significant contributions to our understanding of interpersonal processes is the classic book *Pragmatics of Human Communication* (1967) by Watzlawick, Beavin, and Jackson. The concepts presented here are primarily drawn from this important book on communication and have been updated by the recent research studies of Janet Beavin Bavelas (1992).

Concept 1: All nonverbal communication is meaningful.

This concept helps us to realize that there is no such thing as *not* communicating when we are in the presence of another because all nonverbal communication carries a message (Watzlawick, Beavin, & Jackson, 1967). In personal communication with Dr. Janet Beavin Bavelas, and in her 1992 publication, she states that she now makes a distinction between nonverbal behavior (NVB) and nonverbal communication (NVC). NVC is viewed as a subset of NVB. With NVB there is an "inference-making observer," whereas with NVC, there is a "communicating person" (encoder). In the 1967 text, the concept was presented that all NVB is meaningful.

A significant component of this concept is context. Behavior is only relevant and meaningful when the immediate context is considered. A mother complains to the CHN that she has been experiencing insomnia for 2 months and finds herself very irritable due to the prolonged sleep deprivation. This behavior of the mother needs to be understood in her immediate context. On further exploration, the nurse discovered that this mother has a child on an apnea monitor and that the father sleeps soundly. Therefore, the mother's insomnia will be understood and treated more fully by the CHN with this additional context information.

Concept 2: All communication has two major channels for transmission: digital and analogic.

Digital communication is what is normally referred to as verbal communication. It consists of the actual content of the message, or the brute facts. For example, a mother may say, "I have lost 15 pounds this past month" or a 10-year-old girl may say, "I can now give myself my own insulin." However, when the analogic communication is also taken into account, the meaning of these facts may change dramatically.

Analogic communication not only consists of the usual types of nonverbal communication such as body posture, facial expression, and tone, but also music, poetry, and painting. It can be seen that a woman who presents herself as quite obese and states that she has lost 15 pounds in a month will give a more positive message, both digitally and analogically, than a woman who is very emaciated and states that she has lost 15 pounds.

In discussing the two channels of communication, we do not wish to imply that there are separate verbal and nonverbal channels dedicated to different uses. Bavelas (1992) has accumulated "a great deal of data in favor of an alternative, 'whole message model' in which verbal and nonverbal acts are completely integrated and often interchangeable" (p. 23). Based on our clinical experience, we agree with her research experience that nonverbal communication is an integrated part of language.

If there are discrepancies between the analogic and digital communication (e.g., a teenager says, "It doesn't bother me" about being in a cumbersome cast, but the teenager's eyes are filled with tears), then the analogic mode of communicating is considered the more pertinent to the nurse's observing eye. To the teenager's friend, the digital communication may be the most relevant.

Concept 3: A dyadic relationship has varying degrees of symmetry and complementarity.

These terms are very useful in identifying typical family interaction patterns. Jackson (1973) discussed these terms:

> A complementary relationship consists of one individual giving and the other receiving. In a complementary relationship, the two people are of unequal status in the sense that one appears to be in the superior position, meaning that he initiates action and the other appears to follow that action. Thus the two individuals fit together or complement each other. The most obvious and basic complementary relationship would be the mother and infant. A symmetrical relationship is one between two people who behave as if they have equal status. Each person exhibits the rights to initiate action, criticize the other, offer advice and so on. This type of relationship tends to become competitive; if one person mentions that he has succeeded in some endeavor the other person mentions that he has succeeded in an equally important endeavor. The individuals in such a relationship emphasize their equality or their symmetry with each other. The most obvious symmetrical relationship is a pre-adolescent peer relationship. (p. 189)

Whether a relationship is complementary or symmetrical is no indicator of the health of the relationship. Rather, it is the context that is important in determining the health of the relationship. There are many situations in which complementary and symmetrical relationships are appropriate and healthy. For example, an employee needs to be able to take a one-down position to the employer most of the time. If the employee is unable to do this, it could result in increasing conflict and eventually a relationship that is predominantly symmetrical. This symmetrical escalation could have the end result of the employer dismissing the employee or the employee quitting on unpleasant terms. An example of a healthy symmetrical relationship could be two individuals involved in a tennis match.

In family relationships, the *predominance* of complementary *or* symmetrical behavior usually results in problems. Couples, especially, need to experience a balance between situations and experiences where symmetry and complementarity exist. Parent-child relationships, however, need to experience a gradual shift from a predominant complementary relationship as the child moves into the teenage and young adult years.

> **Concept 4:** All communication consists of two levels: content and relationship.

Communication consists not only of what is being said (content) but also of information that defines the nature of the relationship between those interacting. For example, a father may say to his son, "Come over here son, I want to tell you something," or "*Get* over here, I've got something to *tell you!*" These statements are similar in content, but each implies a very different relationship. The first statement could be viewed as part of a loving relationship; the second statement implies a conflictual relationship.

CHANGE THEORY

The process of change is a fascinating phenomenon, and a variety of ideas exist about what constitutes change in family systems. An extensive review of the literature is synthesized and presented with the most profound and salient points followed by our own beliefs about change and the conditions that affect the change process.

Systems of relationships appear to possess a tendency toward progressive change (Bateson, 1979). However, there is a French proverb that states, "the more something changes the more it remains the same." This beautifully highlights the dilemma nurses frequently face in working with families. The nurse must learn to accept the challenge of the paradoxical relationship between persistence (stability) and change. Maturana (1978) explains the recursiveness of change and stability this way: change is an alteration in the family's structure that occurs as compensation for perturbations and has the purpose of maintaining structure (i.e., stability). Change itself is experienced as a perturbation to the system so that change generates further change and also stability (Maturana, 1978). A change in state is seen as behavior, and therefore differences in family interactional patterns must be explored. Changes in behavior may or may not be accompanied by insight. However, "the most profound and sustaining change will be that which occurs within the family's belief system (cognition)" (Wright & Watson, 1988, p. 425).

Watzlawick, Weakland, and Fisch (1974) suggest that persistence and change need to be considered together despite their opposing natures. They have offered a widely accepted notion of change and have suggested that there are two different types or levels of change. One type they refer to as change occurring within a given system that itself remains unchanged. In other words, the system itself remains unchanged while its elements or parts undergo some type of change. This type of change is referred to as *first-order change*. It is a change in quantity, not quality. First-order change involves using the same problem-solving strategies over and over again. Each new problem is approached mechanically. If a solution to the problem is difficult to find, more old strategies are used and are usually more vigorously applied. An example of first-order change is the learning of a new behavioral strategy to deal with a misbehaving child. A parent who formerly disciplined his child by restricting the child's television watching is said to have undergone first-order change when he now limits the child's spending money.

The second type of change is one whose occurrence changes the system itself. This type of change is referred to as second-order change. *Second-order change* is thus a "change of change." It appears that the French proverb is only applicable to first-order change. With regard to second-order change, there are actual changes in the rules governing the system and, therefore, the system is transformed structurally and/or communicationally. It is also important to note that second-order change is always in the nature of a discontinuity or logical jump and tends to be sudden and radical. This type of change represents a quantum jump in the system to a different level of functioning. Second-order change can be said to occur when parents begin to treat their 16-year-old as an adolescent instead of a child.

Watzlawick, Weakland, and Fisch (1974) also refer to the most obvious source of change. This is *spontaneous* change, by which they mean the type of problem resolution that occurs in daily living without the input of professionals or sophisticated theories.

Hoffman (1980) offers another viewpoint of change and suggests that families, similar to other complex systems, do *not* change in a smooth unbroken line but in discontinuous leaps. She quotes Platt as suggesting that change takes the form of a transformation or a sudden appearance of more functionally organized patterns that did not exist before.

Bateson (1979) offers one of the most thought-provoking statements with regard to change when he suggests that we are almost always unaware of changes. He suggests that changes in our social interactions and in our environment around us are occurring dramatically and constantly but that we become accustomed to the "new state of affairs before our senses can tell us that it is new" (p. 98). Bateson further offers the idea that with regard to the perception of change, the mind can only receive news of difference. Therefore, change can be observed, as Bateson (1979) states, as "difference which occurs across time" (p. 452). These ideas concur with those of

Maturana and Varela (1992), who offer the idea that change is occurring in humans from moment to moment. Such change is either triggered by interaction(s) or pertubations coming from the environment in which the system exists or is a result of the system's own internal dynamics.

Our own view of change in family work has been drawn from some of the above authors as well as from our own clinical experience in working with families. In summary, we believe with Bateson, Maturana, and Varela that change *is* constantly evolving in families and that frequently we are unaware of change. This is the type of continuous or spontaneous change that occurs with everyday living and progression through individual and family stages of development. These changes may or may not occur with professional input.

We also believe that major transformations of an entire family system can occur as a result of or be precipitated by major life events or by interventions from professionals such as nurses. Change within a family may occur within the cognitive, affective, or behavioral domain, but change in any one domain will have an impact on the other domains. Interventions can be aimed at any or all of the three domains. Interventions are discussed further in Chapter 4 when the Calgary Family Intervention Model is presented.

We disagree with Lancaster (1982) that it is possible through the use of systems conceptualization "to predict the consequences of change within any part of a system by examining the interaction and boundaries of the system members" (p. 25). We believe that it is impossible to know what interventions result in what changes and, therefore, it is impossible to predict outcome or the type of change that will occur within families.

However, an important role for the nurse (operating from a systems perspective) is to carefully observe the connections between systems (Lancaster, 1982). To effect change within the original system (e.g., individual), it is necessary to intervene at the metalevel (e.g., family system). In other words, if the nurse wishes to effect change within a family system, the nurse needs to be able to maintain a metaposition to the family. However, if a problem arises between the nurse and the family (e.g., nurse-family system), then this problem will need to be resolved at a higher level, preferably by a supervisor, who can examine the problem from a further metaposition.

Concept 1: Change is dependent on the perception of the problem.

In a now famous statement, Korzybski proclaimed that "the map is not the territory." In other words, the name is different from the thing named and the description is different from what is described. In applying this to family interviewing, our "mapping" of a particular situation or our perception of a problem follows from how we as nurses choose to see it. Keeney (1982) has suggested that "the punctuating or map is in that sense entirely made up (or inherited) by biological constraints and learned by cultural tradition" (1982, p. 157). We very much agree with Keeney that how we perceive a particular problem has profound implications for how we will intervene and, thus, how change will occur and whether it will be effective.

> Viewing problem behavior not in isolation but in relation to its immediate context—the behavior of other family members—means more than just a specific change of viewpoint, important as that is. This change exemplifies a general shift in epistemology from a search for linear cause and effect change to a cybernetic or systems viewpoint— the understanding and explanation of any selected bit of behavior in terms of its place in a wider, ongoing, organized system of behavior, involving feedback and reciprocal reinforcement throughout. (Fisch, Weakland, & Segal, 1982, pp. 8–9)

One of the most common traps for nurses working with families is to accept one family member's perception as the "truth" or to decide who is "right." Of course there is no one truth or reality or perhaps it is more accurate to say that there are as many truths or realities as there are members in the family (Maturana & Varela, 1992). The important task for the nurse is to accept all family members' perceptions and offer the family another view of their problems. Individual family members draw forth their own reality of a situation based on their history of interactions with persons throughout their lives and their genetic history (Maturana & Varela, 1992). Maturana, in an interview with Simon (1985), offered an even more radical idea with regard to different family members' perceptions.

> Systems theory first enabled us to recognize that all the different views presented by the different members of a family had some validity. But systems theory implied that these were different views of the same system. What I am saying is different. I am *not* saying that the different descriptions that the members of a family make are different views of the *same* system. I am saying that there is no one way which the system is; that there is no absolute, objective family. I am saying that for each member there is a different family; and that each of these is absolutely valid. (p. 36)

Whereas Maturana and Varela (1992) emphasize that human systems "draw forth" reality, constructivists, be they radical constructivists (von Glaserfeld, 1984) or social constructionists, emphasize that reality is constructed or invented (Watzlawick, 1984). One example of the constructivist view from Furth (1987) is that "[the world] is patently not a fixed reality and even less a particular physical environment, but most definitely a world of ever-changing individual constructions, or better . . . a world of social co-constructions" (p. 86).

We concur that there are indeed very different yet valid perceptions of problems. However, as nurses, we are part of a larger societal system and thus are bound by moral, legal, cultural, and societal norms that require us to act in accordance with these norms regarding illegal or dangerous behaviors (Wright, Watson, & Bell, 1990).

If a nurse does not conceptualize human problems from a systems/cybernetics perspective, then the nurse's perceptions of problems will be based on a completely *different* conception of reality due to *different* theoretical assumptions. We wish to emphasize *different* theoretical assumptions as opposed to more correct or "right" views of problems.

Concept 2: Change is dependent on context.

Efforts to promote change in a family system must always take into account the important variable of context. Interventions must be planned with sufficient knowledge of contextual constraints and resources. Nurses need to be aware of their position in the healthcare delivery system vis-à-vis the family. For example, are other professionals involved with the family and if so, what is their role with the family? How does this differ from the nurse's role and how are the nurse and family influenced by and influencing the context in which they find themselves?

Imber Coppersmith (1983) and Imber-Black (1991) present a thoughtful analysis of the place of family therapy in the homeostasis of larger systems. She offers that larger systems (e.g., school, mental health agency, hospital, and public service delivery system) frequently impose certain "rules" on families that ultimately maintain the larger system's homeostasis. The first "rule" she suggests is the rule of linear blame. That is, institutions tend to blame families for difficulties (e.g., unmotivated family) and tend to make referrals for family treatment in order to "cure" the family. This is a process similar to that which families use in sending the identified patient to be "cured."

A second "rule" that Imber Coppersmith (1983) identified as maintaining homeostasis in larger systems is the rule of overinvolvement with clients. Because members of some larger systems, particularly hospital staff, become intensely involved in a patient or family member's life, they frequently have a tendency to go beyond the immediate concerns. The end result is that patients in hospitals and their families find themselves overindulged with services that frequently usurp the family's own resources. This then places the family members in a one-down position in terms of articulating what *they* perceive their present needs to be. When a nurse decides or is asked to complete a family assessment, the nurse may become one more irritant in the life of this family and can be hamstrung before even beginning, due to the number of professionals involved. Therefore, this is another reason why nurses should carefully assess the larger context in which the family and the staff find themselves. In some of these cases, the more serious problem is at the interface of the family with other professionals rather than *within* the family itself. Thus, interventions would need to be targeted at the family-professional system *before* addressing problems at the family system level.

The third "rule" Imber Coppersmith (1983) presents is the rule of undefined leadership. In this situation, families may find themselves in a larger system, such as an outpatient drug assessment and treatment clinic. Families may receive varying ideas on how to deal with a particular problem (e.g., cocaine addiction) depending on whether they are seen at the clinic, at home, or in a class. Usually this occurs because no one clinic or educational program offered within a hospital setting has any more decision-making power than any other regarding a particular family. "In short order, client families may find themselves in a situation quite similar to that of a child whose parents cannot agree" (Imber Coppersmith, 1983, p. 221).

The final "rule" offered by Imber Coppersmith (1983) is the rule of dysfunctional triads. This rule states that conflicts between larger systems, or between families and larger systems, that are unacknowledged or unresolved result in dysfunctional triads prohibiting health behavior. For example, if the family wishes to send their adolescent to a drug rehabilitation center, but the nurse and rehab director have been in conflict over rehab policies, then the family is placed in a situation where pressure from the larger system (nurse/rehab director) leads them to align or take sides with *either* the nurse or rehab director.

Therefore, in the assessment of a family, the nurse must be cognizant of the family's relationship to larger or suprasystems. We agree with Imber-Black (1988), who states that the "seemingly intractable problems between a family and larger systems may be following a pattern that, never recognized, rigidly prescribes roles for everyone involved. For generations a family may present similar problems and grapple with similar nonsolutions" (p. 9). How the family is being influenced by and is influencing its involvement with these suprasystems is important information. Otherwise, change within a family can be thwarted, sabotaged, or impossible if the issue of context is not addressed.

Concept 3: Change is dependent on coevolving goals for treatment.

Change requires that goals be coevolved between nurses and families within a realistic time frame. Frequently, one of the main reasons for failure in working with families is the setting of unrealistic or inappropriate goals. What the nurse is able to achieve, in large part, depends on the nurse's own competence and context of treatment. Frank and open discussions with family members regarding treatment goals can often avoid misunderstanding and disappointments on both sides.

Because one of the primary goals in family intervention is to change or alter the family's view of the problem, nurses can assist family members to search for alternative behavioral, cognitive, and affective responses to problems. Therefore, one of the goals of the nurse is to help the family discover its own solutions to its problems.

The task of setting specific goals for treatment is accomplished in collaboration with the family. Part of the assessment process is to identify which problems the family is most concerned with at present and what changes they would like to see in relation to these problems. This then provides the baseline for the goals of family interviews and becomes the therapeutic contract.

Contracts with families can be either verbal or written. In our own clinical practice and in the practice of our nursing students, we normally make verbal contracts with families stating which specific problems will be tackled during what specified period of time or number of sessions. At the end of that period, progress is evaluated and either the family is terminated or, if further therapeutic work is required, a new contract made.

In most instances, clear goals will be set with families in the form of a contract with verbal commitments made by family members to work on the problems outlined. At conclusion of the contract, evaluation should consist of assessing changes in the family system in addition to changes in the identified patient.

In summary, family assessment and intervention is often more effective and successful if based on clear therapeutic goals. However, it is very uncommon for families to come to family interviews with the understanding that *family* change is required. Therefore, in addition to goal-setting, the nurse must help the family to obtain a different view of its problems. First, the nurse needs to engage the family. This can most easily be accomplished by focusing on the presenting problem *first* and the changes the family desires in relation to it. More information about goal setting is given in Chapter 7.

Concept 4: Understanding alone does not lead to change.

Changes in family work rarely occur by increasing a family's understanding of problems but rather through changes in beliefs and behavior. Too often, health professionals engaged in family work have the assumption that *understanding* a problem will bring about a solution by the family. From a systems perspective, however, we believe the solutions to problems come about as beliefs about problems and patterns change, whether or not this is accompanied by insight.

There has been a tendency within nursing that in order to solve a problem one has to understand its *"why."* Thus, good-intentioned nurses spend many hours attempting to obtain masses of data (usually historical) that will lead them to understand the "why" of a problem. Often, the patient and/or family will encourage the nurse in this quest and even participate in it. For example, patients might ask: "Why did I have my heart attack?" "Why won't my young adult son give up crack?" or "Why did my wife have to die so young?" We strongly *discourage* searching for the "why" answers because we do not believe that this is a precondition for change but rather steers one away from effective efforts at change. We strongly encourage that the prerequisite or precondition for change is not understanding the *why* of a situation but rather understanding the *what!* Therefore, we recommend nurses ask, "*What* is the effect of the father's heart attack on him and on his family?" "*What* are the implications of the father's heart attack on his employment?" These serve a much more useful purpose in paving the way for possible interventions than spending time on the "why's" of situations.

"Why" questions seem to be entrenched in psychoanalytic roots that bring forth psychopathologies. This is not congruent with a systems/cybernetic foundation of understanding family dynamics, which focuses on human problems as interpersonal escalations or dilemmas. Even if on occasion the "why" of a problem *is* understood, this understanding rarely contributes to the problem's solution. Therefore, it is more useful to explore what is being *done* here and now to perpetuate the problem and what can be done here and now to effect a change (Watzlawick, Weakland, & Fisch, 1974). We need to avoid the search for causes, as we then are invited to view problems from a linear rather than a systemic perspective. In other words, we prefer to think that problems reside *between* persons rather than *within* persons.

Concept 5: Change does not necessarily occur equally in all family members.

Remembering the analogy of the mobile presented earlier, imagine the mobile *after* a wind has passed on it. Some pieces would turn or react more rapidly or energetically than others. This is similar to change in family systems in that one family member may begin to respond or change more rapidly than others and by this very process sets up an opportunity for change throughout the rest of the family. This is so because other family members will not be able to respond the same to the family member who is changing and, therefore, there will be a ripple effect of change through the system.

Change is dependent on the recursive (cybernetic) nature of a family system. Therefore, a small intervention can lead to a variety of reactions, with some family members changing more dramatically or more quickly than others.

Concept 6: Facilitating change is the nurse's responsibility.

It is our belief that it is the nurse's responsibility to facilitate change in collaboration with each family. Facilitating change does not presuppose that a nurse can predict the outcome, and the nurse should not be invested in a particular outcome. There is a distinct difference between facilitating change and being an expert in resolving family problems. It is crucial for nurses to avoid making value judgments about how families *should* function. Otherwise, the changes (outcome) in a family system may not be satisfying to the nurse if they are incongruent with how the *nurse* perceives a family should function. It is more important that the *family* is satisfied with its new level of functioning than that the nurse is satisfied.

From time to time, nurses need to evaluate the level or degree of responsibility they feel for treatment. The level of responsibility is out of proportion if the nurse feels more concerned, more worried, or more responsible for family problems than do the families themselves. The opposite response can be detachment or a lack of concern or responsibility by the nurse for facilitating change within families. Both of these extreme responses are indicators for obtaining clinical supervision.

How much change nurses should expect themselves to be able to facilitate in family work depends on their own competence, the context of family treatment, and the response of the family. Nurses need to be cognizant that they are not change agents; they cannot and do not change anyone (Wright & Levac, 1992). Changes in family members are determined by their own biopsychosocial structures, not by others (Maturana & Varela, 1992). Therefore, it is the nurse's responsibility to facilitate a context for change.

Concept 7: Change can be due to a myriad of causes.

Change is influenced by so many different variables that most often it is difficult to know what *specifically* precipitated or triggered the change. It is not always a result of some well thought out intervention. Frequently, it can be the result of the method of inquiry into family problems. Asking interventive questions (Chapter 4) may in and of itself promote change. It is more important to attribute change to the family than to concern oneself about what the *nurse* did to create change (Chapter 9). To search for or take undue credit for change is inappropriate at this stage of our knowledge of the change process in families.

CONCLUSIONS

Nursing is striving to base care of families on solid and clinically useful theories. In increasing their theoretical competency, nurses are assuring families of more complete and comprehensive care. The more theoretically competent nurses become, the more they will feel rewarded in their clinical work with families.

REFERENCES

Allmond, B. W., Buckman, W., & Gofman, H. F. (1979). *The family is the patient.* St. Louis: C. V. Mosby.

Barker, P. (1981). *Basic family therapy.* Baltimore: University Park Press.

Bateson, G. (1979). *Mind and nature.* New York: E. P. Dutton.

Bavelas, J. B. (1992). Research into the pragmatics of human communication. *Journal of Strategic and Systemic Therapies, 11*(2), 15–29.

Becvar, D. S., & Becvar, R. J. (1988). *Family therapy: A systemic integration.* Boston: Allyn & Bacon.

Beer, S. (1974). Cybernetics. In H. von Foerester (Ed.), *Cybernetics of cybernetics* (pp. 2–3). Urbana, IL: Biological Computer Laboratory, University of Illinois.

Chin, R. (1977). The utility of system models and developmental models for practitioners. In J. P. Reihl & Sister C. Roy (Eds.), *Conceptual models for nursing practice* (pp. 46–63). New York: Appleton-Century-Crofts.

Fisch, R., Weakland, J. H., & Segal, L. (1982). *The tactics of change.* San Francisco: Jossey-Bass.

Furth, H. G. (1987). *Knowledge as desire: An essay on Freud and Piaget.* New York: Columbia University Press.

Hoffman, L. (1980). The family life cycle and discontinuous change. In B. Carter & M. McGoldrick (Eds.), *The family cycle: A framework for family therapy* (pp. 53–68). New York: Gardner Press.

Imber-Black, E. (1988). *Families and larger systems: A therapist's guide through the labyrinth.* New York: Guilford Press.

Imber-Black, E. (1991). The family-larger-system perspective. *Family Systems Medicine, 9*(4), 371–396.

Imber Coppersmith, E. (1983). The place of family therapy in the homeostasis of larger systems. In M. Aronson & R. Wolberg (Eds.), *Group and family therapy: An overview* (pp. 216–227). New York: Brunner/Mazel.

Jackson, D. (1973). Family interaction, family homeostasis and some implications for conjoint family psychotherapy. In D. Jackson (Ed.), *Therapy, communication and change* (4th ed, pp. 185–203). Palo Alto, CA: Science & Behavior Books.

Keeney, B. (1982). What is an epistemology of family therapy? *Family Process, 21,* 153–168.

Keeney, B. (1983). *Aesthetics of change.* New York: Guilford Press.

Lancaster, J. (1982). Systems theory and the process of change. In J. Lancaster & W. Lancaster (Eds.), *The nurse as a change agent* (pp. 24–28). St. Louis: C. V. Mosby.

Maturana, H. (1978). Biology of language: The epistemology of reality. In G. Millar and E. Lenneberg (Eds.), *Psychology and biology of language and thought* (pp. 27–63). New York: Academic Press.

Maturana, H., & Varela, F. (1980). *Autopoiesis and cognition: The realization of the living.* Dordrecht, Holland: D. Reidl.

Maturana, H., & Varela, F. (1992). *The tree of knowledge: The biological roots of human understanding.* Boston: Shambhala.

Ranson, D. C. (1984). Random notes: The patient is not a dirty window. *Family Systems Medicine, 2*(2), 230–233.

Selvini-Palazzoli, M., Boscolo, L., Cecchin, G., & Prata, G. (1978). A ritualized prescription in family therapy: Odd days and even days. *Journal of Marriage and Family Counseling, 4*(3), 3–9.

Simon, R. (1985, May/June). Structure is destiny: An interview with Humberto Maturana. *Family Therapy Networker,* pp. 32–43.

Tomm, K. (1980). Towards a cybernetic-systems approach to family therapy at the University of Calgary. In D. S. Freeman (Ed.), *Perspectives on family therapy* (pp. 3–18). Toronto: Butterworth.

Tomm, K. (1981). Circularity: A preferred orientation for family assessment. In A. S. Gurman (Ed.), *Questions and answers in the practice of family therapy* (Vol. 1, pp. 874–887). New York: Brunner/Mazel.

Tomm, K. (1984). One perspective on the Milan systemic approach: 2. Description of session format, interviewing style and interventions. *Journal of Marital and Family Therapy, 10*(3), 253–271.

Varela, F. J. (1979). *Principles of biological autonomy.* New York: Elsevier.

von Bertalanffy, L. (1968). *General systems theory: Foundations, development, applications.* New York: George Braziller.

von Bertalanffy, L. (1972). The history and status of general systems theory. In G. Klir (Ed.), *Trends in general systems theory.* New York: John Wiley & Sons.

von Bertalanffy, L. (1974). General systems theory and psychiatry. In S. Arieti (Ed.), *American handbook of psychiatry* (pp. 1095–1117). New York: Basic Books.

von Foerester, H. (1974). Notes for an epistemology of living things. In E. Morin & M. Piatelli (Eds.), *L'unite de l'homme.* Paris: Seuil.

von Glaserfeld, E. (1984). An introduction to radical constructivism. In P. Watzlawick (Ed.), *The invented reality: Contributions to constructivism* (pp. 17–40). New York: W. W. Norton.

Watzlawick, P. (Ed.). (1984). *The invented reality: Contributions to constructivism.* New York: W. W. Norton.

Watzlawick, P., Beavin, J. H., & Jackson, D. D. (1967). *Pragmatics of human communication.* New York: W. W. Norton.

Watzlawick, P., Weakland, J., & Fisch, R. (1974). *Change: Principles of problem formulation and problem resolution.* New York: W. W. Norton.

Wright, L. M., & Levac, A. M. (1992). The non-existence of non-compliant families: The influence of Humberto Maturana. *Journal of Advanced Nursing, 17,* 913–917.

Wright, L. M., & Watson, W. L. (1988). Systemic family therapy and family development. In C. J. Falicov (Ed.), *Family transitions: Continuity and change over the life cycle* (pp. 407–430). New York: Guilford Press.

Wright, L. M., Watson, W. L., & Bell, J. M. (1990). The Family Nursing Unit: A unique integration of research, education and clinical practice. In J. M. Bell, W. L. Watson, & L. M. Wright (Eds.), *The cutting edge of family nursing* (pp. 95–109). Calgary, Alberta: Family Nursing Unit Publications.

THE CALGARY FAMILY ASSESSMENT MODEL

The Calgary Family Assessment Model (CFAM) is an integrated, multidimensional framework based on the systems, cybernetics, communication, and change theoretical foundations. It has received wide recognition since the first edition of this book in 1984. CFAM has been adopted by many faculties and schools of nursing in North America. It has been referenced frequently in the literature and by contributors in the three-volume Family Nursing Series: *Families and Life-Threatening Illness* (Leahey & Wright, 1987a), *Families and Chronic Illness* (Wright and Leahey, 1987), and *Families and Psychosocial Problems* (Leahey & Wright, 1987b). We originally adapted a family assessment framework developed by Tomm and Sanders (1983). However, this present CFAM has now been substantially revised and embellished in this chapter.

CFAM consists of three major categories:

1. Structural
2. Developmental
3. Functional

Each category contains several subcategories. It is important for *each* nurse to decide which subcategories are relevant and appropriate to explore and assess with *each* family at *each* point in time. That is, not all subcategories need to be assessed at a first meeting with a family, and some subcategories need never be assessed. If nurses use too many subcategories, they may become overwhelmed by all the data. If they assess two few, they may have a distorted view of the family situation.

It is useful to conceptualize the three assessment categories (structural, developmental, and functional) and the many subcategories as a branching diagram (Fig. 3–1).

As the nurse uses the subcategories on the right of the branching

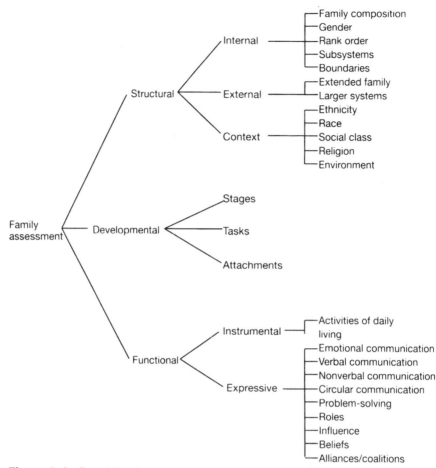

Figure 3–1. *Branching diagram of CFAM.*

diagram, the nurse collects more and more microscopic data. It is important for the nurse to be able to move back and forth on the diagram to draw together all of the relevant information into an integrated assessment.

In this chapter, each assessment category is discussed separately. Terms are defined and sample questions are proposed for the nurse to ask family members. Various types of assessment questions are presented and examples given. The use of assessment and interventive questions will be discussed in Chapter 4, The Calgary Family Intervention Model (CFIM). Again, we wish to emphasize that not all questions about various subcategories of the model need to be asked at the first interview, and questions about each subcategory are not appropriate for every family. Families are obviously composed of individuals, but the focus of a family assessment is less on the individual and more on the interaction *among* all of the individuals within the family.

STRUCTURAL ASSESSMENT

In assessing a family, the nurse needs to examine its structure, that is, who is in the family, what is the connection among family members vis-à-vis those outside the family, and what is the family's context. Three aspects of family structure can most readily be examined: internal structure, external structure, and context. Each of these dimensions of family structural assessment are addressed separately.

INTERNAL STRUCTURE

This aspect includes five subcategories:

1. Family composition
2. Gender
3. Rank order
4. Subsystem
5. Boundary

Family Composition

This subcategory has many meanings. Terkelson (1980) defines a family as a "small social system made up of individuals related to each other by reason of strong reciprocal affections and loyalties, and comprising a permanent household or (cluster of households) that persists over years and decades" (p. 23). Stuart (1991) concludes that there are five critical attributes to the concept of family:

1. The family is a system or unit.
2. Its members may or may not be related and may or may not live together.
3. The unit may or may not contain children.
4. There is commitment and attachment among unit members that include future obligation.
5. The unit caregiving functions consist of protection, nourishment and socialization of its members. (p. 40).

Using these ideas, the nurse can include the various family forms that are prevalent in society today, such as the biological family of procreation; the nuclear family that incorporates one or more members of the extended family (family of origin); the sole-parent family; the stepfamily; the communal family; or the homosexual couple or family. Designating a group of people with a term such as "couple," "nuclear family," or "single-parent family" specifies attributes of membership, but these distinctions of grouping are not more or less "families" by reason of labeling. Rather, attributes of affection, strong emotional ties, a sense of belonging, and durability of membership determine family composition.

We have found the following definition of family to be most useful in our clinical work: the family is who they say they are. Although we recognize the dominant North American type of separately housed nuclear families, our definition allows us to address the emotional past, present, and anticipated future relationships within the family system. Our definition is based on the family's beliefs about *their* conception of family rather than on who lives in the household.

Changes in family composition are important to note. These changes could be due to the loss of a family member or the addition of a new person. Losses tend to be more severe the more recently they have occurred, the younger family members are when loss occurs, the smaller the family, the greater the numerical imbalance between male and female members of the family resulting from the loss, the greater the number of losses, and the greater the number of prior losses (Toman, 1976). Brown (1988) asserts that serious illness or death of a family member can lead to disruption in the family. The extent of the impact of a death on the family depends on the social and ethnic meaning of death, the history of previous losses, the timing of the death in the life cycle, and nature of the death (Walsh & McGoldrick, 1991). The position and function of the person who died in the family system and the openness of the family system must also be considered. We have found it useful to note the family's losses and deaths during the structural assessment process but do not immediately assume that these losses are of major significance to the family. By taking this stance, we disagree with the position taken by McGoldrick (1991), who asserts that "it is important to track patterns of adaptation to loss as a routine part of family assessment even when it is not initially presented as relevant to chief complaints" (p. 52).

In our clinical practice with families we have found it useful to ask ourselves, Who is in *this* family? Who does the family consider to be "family"?

Questions to Ask the Family. Could you tell me who is in your family? Does anyone else live with you, for example, grandparents, boarders? So, there are yourself and your 60-year-old son—anyone else? Has anyone recently moved out? Is there anyone else who you think of as family who does not live with you? Anyone not related biologically?

Gender

This subcategory is a basic construct, a "fundamental organizing principle of all family systems" (Goldner, 1988, p. 17). Since the first edition of our book, there has been an explosion of interest in the subject of gender. We believe in the constructivist "both/and" position, that is, we view gender as both a universal "realty" operational in hierarchy and power and a reality constructed by ourselves from our particular frame of reference. We recognize gender both as a fundamental basis for all human beings and as an individual premise. Gender is important for nurses to consider because the difference in how males and females experience the world is at the heart of the therapeutic conversation. Often in couple relationships the problems described by men and women include unspoken conflicts between their perceptions of gender—that is, how their family and society tell them that men and women should feel, think, or behave—and their own experiences.

We agree with Sheinberg and Penn (1991), who argue on behalf of the integration of male and female attributes in each person. Human development is a process of increasingly complex forms of relatedness and integration rather than a progression from attachment to separation. Gender is, in our view, a set of beliefs about or expectations of male and female behavior and experiences. These beliefs have been developed by cultural, religious, and familial influences. They are in some ways more important than anatomical differences. Sheinberg and Penn (1991) define maturity as "an alternating of both connections and differentiation within the context of ongoing relationships" (p. 35). This definition supports a developmental model based not solely on male norms but rather representative of both genders.

In our clinical supervision with nurses we have found it useful to have them consider their own ideas about masculinity and femininity. For example, as a woman, how do you believe you should behave toward men? How do you expect them to behave toward you? Do you believe men should express emotion? Should women feel entitled to put themselves first? To feel competitive?

Questions to Ask the Family. What effect did your parents' ideas have on your own ideas of masculinity and femininity? If your parents had had different ideas about male or female behavior, how might it have changed your relationship with them? How might it have changed your relationship with your spouse? Would you like your child to feel differently than you do about his or her masculinity or femininity? If your arguments with your child were about how to stay connected to each other rather than how to separate, would they be different? If you would show the feelings you keep hidden, would your wife think more or less of you?

Rank Order

This subcategory refers to the position of the children in the family with respect to age and gender. Birth order, gender, and distance in age between siblings are important factors to consider when doing an assessment. Toman (1988) has been a major contributor to research about sibling configuration. His main thesis is the duplication theorem. He asserts that the more new social relationships resemble earlier intrafamilial social relationships the more enduring and successful they are. For example, the marriage between the older brother (of a younger sister) and the younger sister (of an older brother) has good potential for success because the relationships are complementary. If the marriage is between two first-borns, there might be a symmetrical competitive relationship, each one vying for the position of leadership.

McGoldrick and Gerson (1985) suggest that the following factors also influence sibling constellation: the timing of each sibling's birth in the family history, the child's characteristics, the family's idealized "program" for the child, and the parental attitudes and biases regarding sex differences. Although we believe that sibling patterns are important to note, we urge nurses to remember that different child-rearing patterns have also emerged due to the increased use of birth control, the women's movement, and the entry of more women into the workforce. We agree with Simon's (1988) position that sibling position is an organizing influence on the personality but is not a fixed influence. Each new period of life seems to bring a reevaluation of these influences. An individual transfers or generalizes familial experiences to social settings outside the family, such as kindergarten, schools, and clubs. As an individual is influenced by the environment, his or her relationships with colleagues, friends, and spouses are also generally affected. With the passage of time, there are multiple influences on personality organization in addition to sibling constellation.

Prior to meeting with a family, we encourage nurses to hypothesize about the potential influence of rank order on the reason for the family interview. For example, the nurse could ask herself, "If this child is the youngest in the family, could this be influencing the parents' reluctance to allow him to give his own insulin injection?" The nurse could also consider the influence of birth order on motivation, achievement, and vocational choice. For example, is the firstborn child under pressure to achieve academically?

Questions to Ask the Family. How many children do you have? Who is the eldest? How old is he? Who comes next in line? Have there been any miscarriages or abortions?

Subsystem

This subcategory is a term used to label or mark the family system's level of differentiation. A family carries out its functions through its subsystems. Dyads, such as husband-wife or mother-child, can be seen as subsystems. Subsystems can be delineated by generation, sex, interest, or function (Minuchin, 1974).

Each person in the family belongs to several different subsystems. In each, that person has a different level of power and uses different skills. A 65-year-old woman can be a grandmother, mother, wife, and daughter within the same family. An eldest boy child is a member of the sibling subsystem, the male subsystem, and the parent-child subsystem. In each of the subsystems, he behaves according to his position. He has to concede the power that he exerts over his younger brother in the sibling subsystem when he interacts with his stepmother in the parent-child subsystem. The ability to adapt to the demands of different subsystem levels is a necessary skill for each family member.

In our clinical practice we have found it useful to consider whether there are clear generational boundaries present in the family. If there are, does the family find them helpful or not? For example, we ask ourselves whether one child behaves like a parent or a husband surrogate. Is the child a child or is there a surrogate-spouse subsystem? By generating these hypotheses prior to and during the family meeting, we will be able to connect isolated bits of data either to confirm or to negate a hypothesis.

Questions to Ask the Family. Some families have special subgroups; for example, the women do certain things while the men do other things. Are there different subgroups in your family? What effect does it have on your family? If your family were to have more subgroups, what effect do you think that might have? When Mom and Rose Marie stay up at night and talk together about Dad's use of crack, what do the boys do?

Boundary

This subcategory refers to the rule "defining who participates and how" (Minuchin, 1974, p. 53). Family systems and subsystems have boundaries, the function of which is to protect the differentiation of the system or subsystem. For example, the boundary of a family system is defined when a father tells his teenage daughter that her boyfriend cannot move into the household. A parent-child subsystem boundary is made explicit when a mother tells her daughter, "You are not your brother's parent. If he is not taking his medication, I'll discuss it with him."

Boundaries can be diffuse, rigid, or appropriately permeable. As boundaries become diffuse, the differentiation of the family system decreases. For example, family members may become too enmeshed, emotionally close, and "too richly cross-joined" (Ashby, 1969, p. 208). These family members have a heightened sense of belonging to the family at the expense of their individual autonomy. A diffuse subsystem boundary is evident when a child is parentified or given adult responsibilities and power in decision making.

When there are rigid boundaries, the subsystems tend to become disengaged. A husband who rigidly believes that "only wives should visit the elderly," and whose wife agrees with him, can become disengaged from or peripheral to the senior adult-child subsystem. Clear, permeable boundaries, on the other hand, allow for appropriate flexibility. There are rules, but they can be modified. Therefore, family members are neither too enmeshed nor too disengaged.

Boundaries tend to change over time. Boss (1980) suggests that family boundaries become ambiguous "during the process of reorganization after acquisition or loss of a member" (p. 445). This is particularly evident with families experiencing separation or divorce. Burns (1987) suggests that the involuntarily childless couple may experience infertility as a stress of boundary ambiguity; that is, not knowing whether their unconceived child is in or out of the family system. She hypothesizes that as infertile couples attempt to make the transition to parenthood they may experience the desired child as a family member who is psychologically present but physically absent.

Boundary styles can facilitate or constrain family functioning. For example, an immigrant family that moves into a new culture may initially be very protective of its members until it gradually adapts to the cultural milieu. Its boundaries vis-à-vis outside systems will be quite firm and rigid but gradually will become more flexible.

In our clinical supervision with nurses, we encourage them to consider how this family differentiates itself from other families in the neighborhood and in the city. The nurse considers whether there is a parental subsystem, a marital subsystem, a sibling subsystem, and so forth. Are the boundaries clear, rigid, or diffuse? Does the boundary style facilitate or constrain the family?

Questions to Ask the Family. The nurse can infer the boundaries by asking the husband if there is anyone with whom he can talk when he feels stressed by his retirement. The nurse can ask the wife the same question. Whom would you go to if you felt happy? If you felt sad? Would there be anyone in your family opposed to your talking with that person? Who would be most in favor of you talking with that person?

EXTERNAL STRUCTURE

This aspect includes two subcategories:

1. Extended family
2. Larger systems

Extended Family

This subcategory includes the family of origin and the family of procreation as well as the present generation and steprelatives. Multiple loyalty ties to extended family members can be invisible but may be very influential forces in the family structure. How each member sees himself or herself as a separate individual yet part of the "family ego mass" (Bowen, 1978) is a critical structural area for assessment.

In our clinical work we consider whether there are many references to the extended family. How significant is the extended family to the functioning of this particular family? Are they available for support in times of need?

Questions to Ask the Family. Where do your parents live? How often do you have contact with them? What about your brothers and sisters? Which family members do you never see? Which of the relatives are you closest to? Who telephones whom? With what frequency? Who do you ask for help when problems arise in your family? What kind of help do you ask for? Would you be available if they needed your help?

Larger Systems

This subcategory refers to the larger social agencies and personnel with whom the family has meaningful contact. Such larger systems generally include work systems, and for some families they include public welfare, child welfare, foster care, courts, and outpatient clinics. There are also larger systems designed for special populations, such as agencies mandated to provide services to the mentally or physically handicapped or the frail elderly. For many families, engagement with such larger systems is not problematic. Imber-Black (1991) states that some families and larger systems, however, may develop difficult relationships that exert a toll on normative development for family members. Some healthcare professionals in larger systems contribute to families being labeled "multiproblem," "resistant," or "uncooperative." These healthcare professionals limit their perspective to include only the family system rather than taking the more complex perspective that includes the family's relationship to larger systems and multiple helpers.

In our clinical supervision with nurses we encourage them to discover whether the *meaningful system* is the family alone or the family *and* its larger-system helpers. Nurses can ask themselves such questions as, who are the healthcare professionals involved? What is the relationship between the family and the larger-system professionals? How regularly do they interact? Is their relationship symmetrical or complementary? Are the larger systems overconcerned? Overinvolved? Underconcerned? Underinvolved? Is the family blamed for its problems by the larger system? What do the helpers desire for the family? Is the nurse being asked to take responsibility for another system's task? How do the family and helpers define the problem?

Questions to Ask the Family. What agency professionals are involved with your family? How many agencies regularly interact with you? Has your family moved from one healthcare system to another? Who most thinks that your family needs to be involved with these systems? Who most thinks the opposite? Would there be agreement between your definition of the problem and the system's definition of the problem? How about between your definitions of the solution?

CONTEXT

Context is explained as the whole situation or background relevant to some event or personality. Each family system is itself nested within broader systems such as neighborhood, class, region, and country, and is influenced by these systems. Because the context permeates and circumscribes both the individual and the family, its consequences are pervasive. Context includes five subcategories:

1. Ethnicity
2. Race

3. Social class
4. Religion
5. Environment

Ethnicity

This subcategory refers to a concept of a family's "peoplehood" derived from a combination of cultural history, race, and religion. It describes a commonality of conscious and unconscious processes transmitted by the family over generations and usually reinforced by the surrounding community (McGoldrick, 1988a). Ethnicity is an important factor influencing family interaction. We believe that nurses must be aware of the great variety within ethnic groups as well as between ethnic groups. For example, Cheng-Ham (1989) points out that there are three different classifications of immigrant groups. There are those who are second-, third-, or fourth-generation immigrants with ancestors from a foreign country. There are the "recently arrived" immigrant families, of whom some are refugees. There are also those "immigrant-American" families, in which the parents were born in a foreign country and their children were born in the United States. For immigrant families, the impact of cultural adjustment can be seen as a transitional difficulty, with issues such as economic survival, racism, and changes in extended family and support system that need to be addressed. Specific life experiences, such as a college education, financial success in business, or family intermarriage can encourage assimilation into a dominant culture, whereas isolation in a rural area or urban ghetto tends to foster continuity of ethnic patterns.

Ethnic differences in family structure and their implications for intervention can be highlighted (McGoldrick, 1982). For example, Italians in North America usually have strong extended family connections and loyalties. African-Americans tend to have flexible family boundaries and some may include the grandmother in child rearing. Puerto Ricans and members of some Latin American cultures encourage emotionality between relatives and between generations, whereas the Irish in North America have more strictly defined boundaries between generations.

In our clinical work we have found it essential to recognize the infinite variety and lack of stereotype in families from various ethnic groups. Nurses should sensitize themselves to differences in family beliefs and values and be willing to alter their "ethnic filters." We believe it is important for nurses to recognize their own ethnic blind spots and adjust their interventions accordingly. Some questions that we have found useful to ask ourselves include: What is the family's ethnicity? Is their social network from the same ethnic group? Do they find that helpful or not? If the available economic, educational, health, legal, and recreational services were similar to the family's ethnic values, how would our conversation be different?

Questions to Ask the Family. I would like to learn more about your ethnic background. Could you tell me about your ethnic practices regarding illness? How does your ethnicity influence your beliefs about when to consult with health professionals? What does health mean to you? How would you know that you are healthy? How would I know that you are healthy?

Race

This subcategory is a basic construct and not an intermediate variable. Race influences core individual and group identification. It intersects with such mediating variables as class, religion, and ethnicity. Racial attitudes, stereotyping, and discrimination are powerful influences on family interaction and, if left unaddressed, can be negative constraints on the relationship between the family and the nurse. Only recently has the "myth of sameness" (Hardy, 1990) been challenged and the uniqueness of various family forms emphasized. Family clinicians are now starting to appreciate that the variations in family structure and development of African-Americans, Asians, Hispanics, whites, and others are potentially strengths in helping families to function under various economic and social conditions.

In our clinical work with families, we have found it very useful to challenge our own ideas about "the myth of sameness" and to vigorously pursue the differences between and within various racial groups. For example, we ask ourselves how a Jamaican-American family might differ from an African-American family in their beliefs about hospitalization. How might a Vietnamese couple differ from a Japanese couple in their beliefs about whether to institutionalize an aging grandmother?

Questions to Ask the Family. What differences do you notice between, for example, your Hispanic relatives' child-rearing practices and your own? If you and I were the same race, would our conversation be different? How? Would our different type of conversation be more or less likely to assist you in regaining your health?

Social Class

This subcategory shapes educational attainment, income, and occupation. Each class, whether upper-upper, lower-upper, upper-middle, lower-middle, upper-lower, or lower-lower, has its own clustering of values, lifestyles, and behavior that influences family interaction and healthcare practices. For example, middle-class seniors are more likely to help their adult children, whereas working-class older adults are more likely to receive help.

Social class has been referred to as one of the prime molders of the family value and belief system. Hampson, Beavers, and Hulgus (1990) assert that much of the sociological and psychological research has been confounded by social class differences among ethnic groups. We agree and wish to point out additional confounding issues. Because poverty is disproportionately concentrated among racial minorities, many professionals have considered the African-American statistical subgroup to represent the lower-income class and the white statistical subgroup to represent the middle- or upper-income class group. Furthermore, although Hispanics, which includes Mexicans, Puerto Ricans, Cubans, and people from South and Central America, have increased substantially in number to become a sizable minority within the United States, until recently data about marriage and family has excluded them. Such data have generally been limited to blacks (African-Americans) and whites, without taking into account Hispanics or Asians. Much of the literature confounds the effects of race and class, not to mention the "myth of sameness" about families within each race or class.

Just as nursing often has been presented as intercultural, so it has also been presented as interclass and nonpolitical. We believe that many nurses have pursued sickness in families to the exclusion of obtaining the *meaning* people give to events, their day-to-day living standards, access to employment, income, and housing. Social class issues often have been seen to be of little consequence to the "serious talk" about illness. This has enabled nurses to sidestep many class issues associated with inequality and injustice. We agree with Waldegrave (1990) that treatment must take into account the cultural, social, and economic context of the persons seeking help.

We have in our clinical work asked ourselves how the family's social class might be influencing their healthcare beliefs, values, utilization of services, and interaction with us. We have wondered about the intrafamilial differences with respect to class and how these might help or hinder a family coping with, for example, chronic illness.

Questions to Ask the Family. How many moves have you had in the past 5 years? Have the moves had a more positive or negative influence on, for example, your ability to deal with your son's having AIDS? How many schools has your daughter attended? How many hours a week do you work? How does your money situation influence your use of healthcare resources?

Religion

This subcategory influences family values, size, healthcare, and socialization practices. For example, individualism is intricately related to the Protestant work ethic. Community support, on the other hand, is very evident in the Mormon and Jewish religions, which foster intergenerational and intragenerational support. Folk healing traditions that combine health and religious practices are quite common in some ethnic groups. There are some spiritualistic practices in which a medium is a counselor helping to exorcise the spirits causing illness. For example, *espiritistas* or healers can be found in many Cuban and other Latino communities.

As nursing has evolved, it has begun to consider spirituality as a hidden and often underused resource in family work. Berenson (1990) writes that "it could be said, spirituality is to conventional religion as systems thinking is to linear, cause and effect thinking" (p. 59). Spirituality stems not so much from institutionalized religious beliefs and practices as from a family's ways of relating to the world. The striking success of Alcoholics Anonymous in making the distinction between spirituality and religion and capitalizing on changes within individuals and families has been acknowledged recently.

In our clinical work we have asked ourselves about the influence of religion and spirituality on the family's healthcare practices. We have noted whether there are signs of religious influence in the home, for example, statues, candles, flags, and religious texts such as the Bible and the Koran.

Questions to Ask the Family. Are you involved with a church, temple, or synagogue? If you had a family problem would you talk with anyone in your church or temple? Are your spiritual beliefs a resource for you? For you and other family members? Who among your family members would be most encouraging of your using your spirituality to help you cope with your life-threatening illness?

Environment

This subcategory encompasses aspects of the larger community, the neighborhood, and the home. Environmental factors such as adequacy of space and privacy and accessibility of schools, day care, recreation, and public transportation influence family functioning. These are especially relevant for older adults, who are more likely to remain in a poor environment even if it has become dangerous to live there. Over the past decade we have had to adjust our perceptions of homelessness and come to grips with the idea that families with children are the fastest growing homeless group. Homelessness is neither an urban nor a regional problem, but rather one that is pervasive in North America.

In our clinical work with families, we have asked ourselves and the nurses with whom we work to assess whether the home is adequate for the number of people living there. Does our perception differ from the family's? What health and other basic services are available within the home? Within the neighborhood? How accessible in terms of distance, convenience, and so forth are transportation and recreation services?

Questions to Ask the Family. What community services does your family use? Are there community services you would like to learn about but do not know how to contact?

STRUCTURAL ASSESSMENT TOOLS

The genogram and the ecomap are two tools that are particularly helpful for the nurse to use in outlining the family's internal and external structures. The genogram is a diagram of the family constellation. The ecomap, on the other hand, is a diagram of the family's contact with others outside of the immediate family. It pictures the important connections between the family and the world. Each is simple to use and requires only a piece of paper and a pen.

These tools have been developed as assessment, planning, and intervention devices. They convey a great deal of information in the form of a visual gestalt. When one considers the number of words it would take to portray the facts thus represented, it becomes clear how simple and useful these tools are.

Genogram

The skeleton of the genogram tends to follow conventional genetic and genealogic charts. It is usual practice to have at least three generations included. Family members are placed on horizontal rows that signify generational lines. For example, a marriage or common-law relationship is denoted by a horizontal line. Children are denoted by vertical lines. Children are rank-ordered from left to right beginning with the eldest child. Each individual is represented. A blank genogram is given in Figure 3–2.

Some authors (McGoldrick & Gerson, 1988) differ slightly in the symbols they use to denote the details of the genogram. The symbols in Figure 3–3, however, are generally agreed on.

Inside the square or circle should be noted the person's name and age. Outside the symbol, significant data (for example, travels a lot, depressed, overinvolved in work, and so forth) should be noted. If a family member has died, the year of his or her death is indicated above the square or circle. When the symbol for miscarriage is used, the sex of the child should be identified if it is known.

A sample of a nuclear and an extended family genogram is given in Figure 3–4.

Alfred Ryan, age 47, has been married to Joan, age 35, since 1977. They have two children: Donna, age 14, in grade 8 and Michael, age 7, who is repeating grade 1. Alfred is employed as a parks department foreman

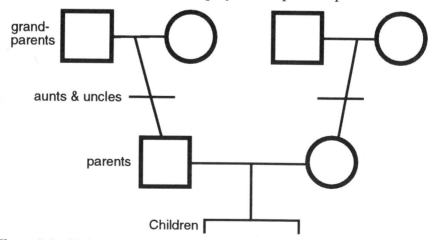

Figure 3–2. Blank genogram. (From McGoldrick and Gerson [1988], with permission.)

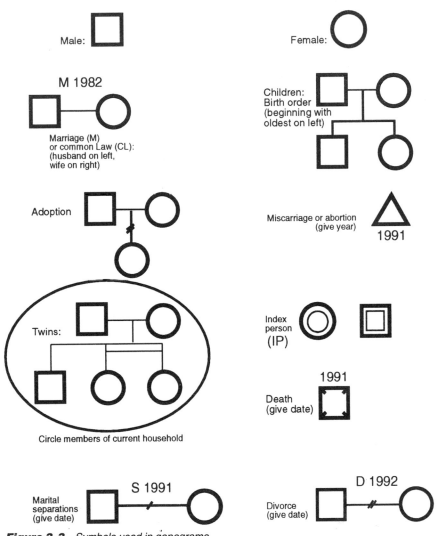

Figure 3–3. Symbols used in genograms.

and Joan refers to him as "alcoholic." Joan is a homemaker and states she has been "depressed" for several years. Both of Alfred's parents are deceased. His father died in 1990 and his mother in 1989 of a stroke. Alfred's older brother also has a drinking problem. The young Michael was named for his grandfather Michael. Joan's mother, Grace, age 54, has arthritis, which has been getting progressively worse since her husband died in 1985. Joan has two older sisters and a brother.

How to Use the Genogram. At the beginning of the interview, the nurse

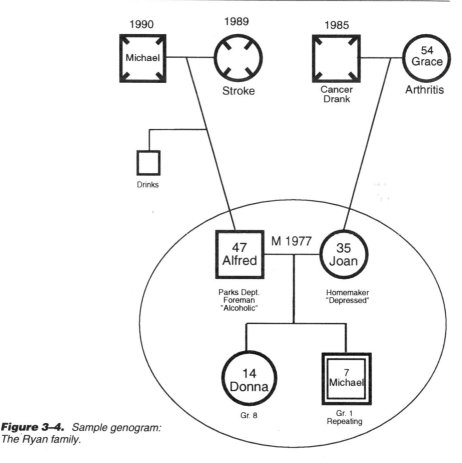

Figure 3–4. Sample genogram: The Ryan family.

informs the family that they will be having a conversation so that she can gain an overview of the family situation, background, and relationships. The nurse can then use the structure of the genogram to discern the family's internal and external structures as well as context. Thus, she gains an understanding of the family's composition and boundaries.

Initially, the nurse starts out with a blank sheet of paper and draws a line or circle for the first person in the family to whom she directs a question.

Nurse: Hilda, you said you were 23, and Hans, how old are you?
Hans: Thirty-four.
Nurse: How long have you been married?
Hans: This time or the first time?
Nurse: This time. And then the first time.
Hans: Just 2 years for Hilda and me.
Nurse: And the first time?
Hans: Ten years for the first one.
Nurse: And Hilda, have you been married before?

Hilda: (*Laughs nervously*) I'm only 23.

Nurse: Sure, it's just that many people have lived together in common-law marriages or have been married when they were very young.

Hilda: No. I lived with my parents till I met Hans.

Nurse: Do either of you have children from prior relationships? (*Turns to both Hans and Hilda*)

Hans: Yes, I have two sons.

Hilda: No.

Nurse: In addition to Karine here (*Looks at infant on couch*), do the two of you have any other children?

Hilda: Yes, there's Fred.

Hans: Old stinko, you mean.

Nurse: Old stinko?

Hans: He isn't toilet trained yet.

Nurse: Oh, I see. And he's how old?

Hilda: He's almost 3. I've been trying to train him since I knew I was pregnant with Karine, but he just doesn't seem to want to go.

Nurse: (*Nods*) Mm.

Hans: Yeah, old stinko!

Nurse: And Karine is how many weeks now?

Hilda: She'll be 21 days tomorrow (*Smiles at infant*).

Nurse: Does anyone else live with you?

Hans: No. Her parents live next door.

The nurse now has a rudimentary genogram of the family (Fig. 3–5). The nurse has gathered information that may or may not be significant depending on the way in which the family has responded to various events in the history of their family.

- Fred was conceived prior to the marriage. Fred is unaffectionately called "old stinko" by his father.
- Mother has been trying to train Fred since he was 24 months.

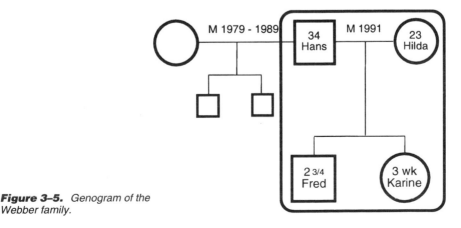

Figure 3–5. Genogram of the Webber family.

- Mother lived with her family of origin prior to the marriage. They live next door.
- Father has been married before and has two sons.

After inquiring about the nuclear family, the nurse can continue to inquire about the extended family. It is generally not very important to go into great detail about these relatives but clinical judgment should prevail. After questions have been asked about the husband's parents and siblings, the nurse should then inquire about the wife's family of origin. What is important is for the nurse to gain an *overview* of the family structure and to try to avoid getting sidetracked or inundated by a large volume of information.

The same question format used for nuclear families is used with stepfamilies—with one exception. It is generally easier to ask one spouse about his or her previous relationships before going on to ask the other spouse about her or his relationships. Again, it is unnecessary to gather specific information on all extended family members. It is useful to draw a circle around the current family members so as to distinguish between the various households. Usually it is easiest to indicate the year of a divorce rather than the number of years ago that it happened. A sample of a genogram showing a stepfamily is given in Figure 3–6.

Bill, age 35, has been living in a common-law marriage since 1989 with Lou, age 33, who is a waitress part-time. Also in the household are

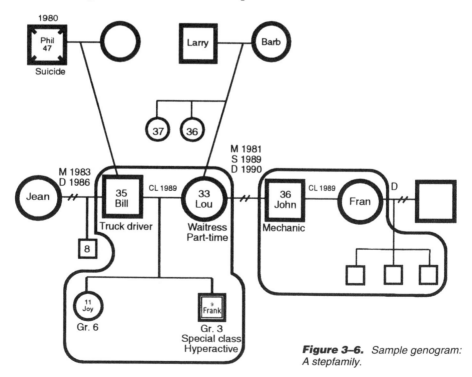

Figure 3–6. *Sample genogram: A stepfamily.*

Lou's two children: Joy, age 11, and Frank, age 9, who is hyperactive and in a special class in grade 3. Bill had been married in 1983 to his first wife, Jean. They were divorced in 1986. Bill and Jean had one son, who is now age 8. Bill was an only child. His father committed suicide in 1980, at the age of 47. His mother is still alive. Lou is the youngest of three daughters, and both her parents are living. Lou was married in 1981 to John, separated in 1989, and divorced in 1990. John, age 36, is a mechanic who is presently living in a common-law marriage with Fran and her three sons.

Most families are extremely receptive to and interested in collaborating with the nurse in completing a genogram. For some, it is the first time that they have ever seen a picture of their family life in this manner. Therefore, the nurse needs to be aware that the family may have a reaction to significant events. One family, for example, may express some sensitive material in a very blasé fashion. If divorce is very common in their families of origin, they may not hesitate to discuss their several marriages and those of their siblings. On the other hand, a devout Catholic family may be exquisitely sensitive to observing the nurse write the word "divorce."

Ecomap

Similar to the genogram, the primary value of the ecomap is in its visual impact. The purpose of the ecomap is to depict the family members' contact with larger systems. Hartman (1978) notes:

> The eco-map portrays an overview of the family in their situation; it pictures the important nurturant or conflict-laden connections between the family and the world. It demonstrates the flow of resources, or the lack of and deprivations. This mapping procedure highlights the nature of the interfaces and points to conflicts to be mediated, bridges to be built, and resources to be sought and mobilized. (p. 467)

How to Use the Ecomap. As with the genogram, family members can actively participate in working on the ecomap during the assessment process. A blank ecomap is depicted in Figure 3–7.

The family genogram is placed in the center circle labeled family or household. The outer circles represent significant people, agencies, or institutions in the family's context. The size of the circles is not important. Lines are drawn between the family and the outer circles to indicate the nature of the connections that exist. Straight lines indicate strong connections, dotted lines indicate tenuous connections, and slashed lines indicate stressful relations. The wider the line the stronger the tie. Arrows can be drawn alongside the lines to indicate the flow of energy and resources. Additional circles may be drawn as necessary depending on the number of significant contacts the family has. An ecomap for the Ryan family has been drawn in Figure 3–8.

Alfred, Joan, Donna, and Mike are placed in the center circle. Alfred has strong connections with his workplace, where he is foreman and a union

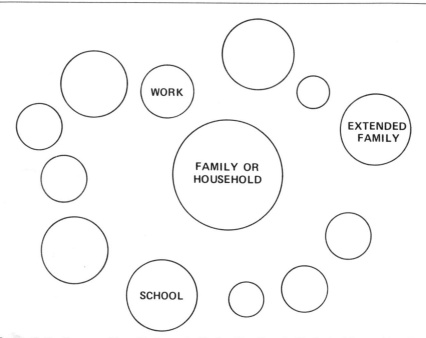

Figure 3–7. *Ecomap. (From Hartman, A: Finding Families: An Ecological Approach to Family Assessment in Adoption. © Copyright 1979. Reprinted by permission of Sage Publications, Inc., Beverly Hills.)*

representative. He has moderately strong bonds with his "drinking buddies." These relationships, however, are stressful for him. Joan's connections are mainly with her mother and the healthcare system. She sees her family physician every week "for nerves" and sees the Community health nurse (CHN) once a week. Joan's mother, Grace, visits Joan every day from 11:00 AM to 10:00 PM. There is a strong connection between Joan and her mother, but Joan says she really "doesn't like Mom coming over so often." Michael has a few friends, most of whom are fire setters. He is in a special class for his learning disability and enjoys both the teacher and the school. Donna is in junior high school, where she maintains an average grade of D. She frequently does not attend school, and when she does attend, she participates little. She spends about 6 hours a day with her boyfriend.

When the CHN completed the ecomap with the Ryan family, Mrs. Ryan commented, "I seem to spend all my time with medical or health people." Mr. Ryan then said, "You're also so busy with your mother that you don't have time for anybody else." The nurse was able to use this information from the ecomap to further discuss with the family the types of relationships they wanted both with those inside their household and with those outside the immediate family.

In summary, the genogram and the ecomap can be used in *all* healthcare settings to increase the nurse's awareness of the whole family and the family's interactions with larger systems and their extended family.

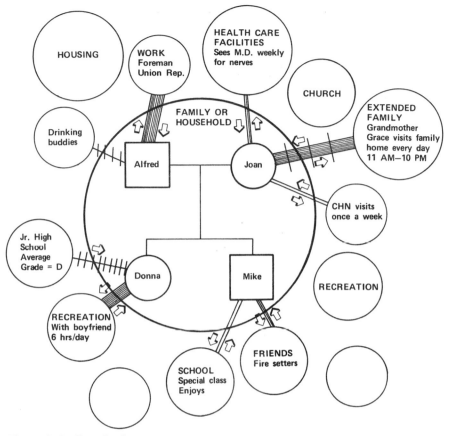

Figure 3–8. *Ryan family ecomap.*

DEVELOPMENTAL ASSESSMENT

In addition to an understanding of the family structure, the nurse requires an understanding of the developmental life cycle for each family. Most nurses are very familiar with stages of child development and the more recent literature in the area of adult development. But what of family development? It is more than the concurrent development at different phases of children and adults who happen to call themselves "family." We concur with Falicov (1988) that "family development is an over-arching concept, referring to *all* transactional evolutionary processes connected with the growth of a family" (p. 13). Such processes as continuity and change related to acute or chronic illness, work or occupational development, relocation, or any other event that significantly alters the texture of family life must be included. Psychological processes such as the development of intimacy, grief reactions, and invisible loyalties are also an integral part of family development. Falicov (1988) writes:

Although there is a regularity and internal logic to many of the processes subsumed under family development . . . each family is different precisely because each can be said to have its own developmental path, which evolves from all the different settings in which development takes place, including each family's construction of its past and present. (p. 13)

In our clinical supervision with nurses, we have found it useful to distinguish between "family development" and "family life cycle." The former emphasizes the *unique* path constructed by a family, whereas the latter refers to the *typical* path most families go through. The typical life cycle events are connected to the comings and goings of family members. For example, most families experience in their life cycle the events of birth, raising of children, departure of children from the household, retirement, and death. Such events generate changes requiring formal reorganization of roles and rules within the family. The life cycle course of families evolves through a generally predictable sequence of stages, despite cultural and ethnic variations. Although individual variations, timing, and coping strategies exist, the biological time clocks and societal expectations for such events as entrance into elementary school and retirement from work are relatively typical.

The early proponents (Duvall, 1977) of the family life cycle developed a four-stage model that was subsequently expanded into an eight-stage model featuring successive stages in the progression of primary marriages. With the increase in various family forms, more complex designs have been created (Hill, 1986; Carter & McGoldrick, 1988). Glick, in 1989, commented that most analyses of the family life cycle begin with a discussion of the first marriage but that it is important also to consider activities that precede the first marriage. This approach reflects in part the increasing delay of marriage and the increasing knowledge about relevant nonmarital behavior that is taking place before young couples marry. As first marriages in the United States generally occur 3 years later than they did a generation ago, more unmarried young adults are cohabitating outside marriage (Glick, 1989a).

There have been a great many changes in the family life cycle just within the past decade. First, there has been an increase in literature discussing families and their developmental phases (e.g., divorce, remarriage, chronic illness, and so forth). Second, there has been an increased awareness of differences in male and female development and the implications of these differences for the family life cycle. Third, there has been a lower birth rate, a longer life expectancy, a change of the roles of women and men, and an increasing divorce and remarriage rate. All of these changes have required a careful rethinking of our assumptions about "normality" and the idea of "family." Hagestad (1988) points out the relationship between demographic changes and alterations in the prevalence, timing, and sequencing of some key family transitions. For example, with people living longer, patterns of family death are now more predictable; grandparenthood is more prevalent and falls into a clearer sequence in the life cycle.

Carter and McGoldrick (1988) believe that the family life cycle perspective views symptoms in relation to normal functioning over time and that "therapy" helps to reestablish the family's developmental momentum. Such family therapists as Haley (1977), Minuchin (1974), and the Milan Group (Selvini, Boscolo, Cecchin, & Prata, 1980) have noted the frequency of symptom appearance with the addition or loss of a family member. These therapists have worked with families that do not move smoothly or automatically from one stage in the family life cycle to another, and they have focused on the stressful transition points between stages. In doing an assessment and in planning interventions, these therapists pay considerable attention to life cycle events as markers of change. Although they differ between themselves, these therapists are similar in seeking to understand the relationship between psychopathology and the family's developmental life cycle stage. For example, Minuchin takes normative expectations into account when validating goals, whereas the Milan systemic group purposefully avoids a normative direction (Wright & Watson, 1988). Carter and McGoldrick (1988) include the impact of transgenerational stress intersecting with current family developmental transitions. They believe if vertical (transgenerational) stress is too high, then a small amount of horizontal (current) stress will lead to great disruption and symptom formation.

In our clinical work with families presenting in various forms and at all stages of development, we have found it useful to adopt Falicov's (1988) ideas about family development. She emphasizes culture and gender relativity rather than universality, transitions rather than stages, dimensions and processes rather than markers, and a resource rather than a deficit orientation. We concur with her idea that a systems approach to family development calls for a dialectical integration of two tendencies: stability and change. The emphasis is on both tendencies rather than one or the other. Change and stability must be addressed simultaneously. We do not find it clinically useful to think of families as "stuck" and unable to bring about change. Rather, we find it clinically useful to look for patterns of continuity, identity, and stability that can be maintained while new behavioral patterns are changing.

We believe there is much evidence to support the position that nurses will find heuristic value in the family development category of CFAM. They should be aware, however, of some of the problems in its indiscriminate adoption and application. We find indefensible such sweeping generalizations as, "The family life cycle is genetically determined," or "The family life cycle is culturally universal." We urge nurses to consider carefully the implication of a family's ethnicity and social class in applying the family development category.

We also caution nurses against *indiscriminately* applying the family development category and overemphasizing *smooth progression*. Contradictions and difficulties inherent in progressing through the life cycle are normal. Families are complex systems that need to deal with many different progressions at once. That is, there are biological, psychological, sociological, and cultural progressions. Tensions and continuing change brought about by contradiction between these progressions are normal. Family life is seldom smooth or bland, but rather is zestful and active. We therefore encourage nurses when using the family development category to have families discuss both their joys and satisfactions and their tensions and stresses.

In addition to delineating stages and tasks implicit in the family life cycle, we have found it useful to assess the attachments between family members. Attachment refers to a relatively enduring, unique emotional tie between two specific persons. Bowlby (1977) notes:

> Affectional bonds and subjective states of a strong emotion tend to go together. . . . Thus many of the most intensive of all emotions arise during the formation, the maintenance, the disruption and renewal of affectional bonds which for that reason are sometimes called emotional bonds. In terms of subjective experience the formation of a bond is described as falling in love, maintaining a bond as loving someone, and losing a partner as grieving over someone. Similarly the threat of loss arouses anxiety and actual loss causes sorrow, while both situations are likely to arouse anger. Finally the unchallenged maintenance of a bond is experienced as a source of security and renewal of a bond as a source of joy. (p. 203)

Although the terms "bonding" and "attachment" are sometimes used to describe different relationships, we have chosen in this book and in our clinical work to make no distinction between these terms. In assessing a

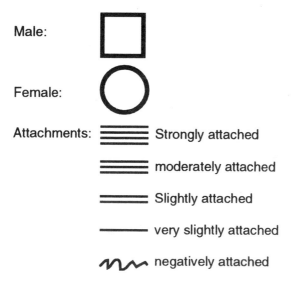

Figure 3–9. Symbols used in attachment diagrams.

family, we tend to pay the most attention to the reciprocal nature of an attachment and the quality of the affectional tie. We illustrate these bonds between family members by drawing attachment diagrams. The symbols used in these diagrams (Fig. 3–9) are similar to those used in the structural assessment diagrams.

In the CFAM developmental category, we discuss family life cycle stages, the emotional process of transition (namely, key principles), and second-order changes—the issues to be dealt with and tasks to be accomplished during each stage. In an effort to emphasize the variability of family development, we discuss five sample types of family life cycles:

1. Middle-class North American family life cycle
2. Divorce and postdivorce family life cycle
3. Remarried family life cycle
4. Comparison of professional and low-income family life cycle stages
5. Adoptive family life cycle

MIDDLE-CLASS NORTH AMERICAN FAMILY LIFE CYCLE

We are grateful to Carter and McGoldrick (1988) for delineating the six stages in the North American middle-class family life cycle (Table 3–1). We highlight the expansion, contraction, and realignment of relationships as entries, exits, and development of family members occur. Although the relationship patterns and family themes may sound familiar, we wish to emphasize that the structure and form of the North American family has changed radically. We believe it is important for nurses to have a positive conceptual frame for what *is*: dual-career families, permanent single-parent households, unmarried couples, homosexual couples, remarried couples, and sole-parent adoptions. Transitional crises should not be thought of as permanent traumas. We believe it is imperative that the use of language that links us to previous stereotypes be dropped. For example, we try to eliminate such phrases as "children of divorce," "working mother," "out-of-wedlock child," "fatherless home," and so forth from the language we use about families.

Stage One: The Launching of the Single Young Adult

In outlining the stages of the middle-class North American family life cycle, we have chosen to start with the stage of "young adults." The primary task of young adults is to come to terms with their family of origin by remaining connected and yet separate, without cutting off or fleeing reactively to a substitute emotional source. The family of origin has a profound influence on who, when, how, and whether the young adult will marry. It is an opportunity for young adults to sort out emotionally what they will take along from the family of origin, what they will leave behind, and what they will establish for themselves as they progress through succeeding stages of the family life cycle. For both men and women, this is a particularly critical phase. Men during this stage sometimes have

TABLE 3–1 MIDDLE-CLASS NORTH AMERICAN FAMILY LIFE CYCLE STAGES AND TASKS

Family Life Cycle Stage	Emotional Process of Transition: Key Principles	Second-Order Changes in Family Status Required to Proceed Developmentally
1. Leaving home: Single young adults	Accepting emotional and financial responsibility for self	1. Differentiation of self in relation to family of origin 2. Development of intimate peer relationships 3. Establishment of self re: work and financial independence
2. The joining of families through marriage: The new couple	Commitment to new system	1. Formation of marital system 2. Realignment of relationships with extended families and friends to include spouse
3. Families with young children	Accepting new members into system	1. Adjusting marital system to make space for child(ren) 2. Joining in childrearing, financial, and household tasks 3. Realignment of relationships with extended family to include parenting and grandparenting roles
4. Families with adolescents	Increasing flexibility of family boundaries to include children's independence and grandparents' frailties	1. Shifting of parent-child relationships to permit adolescent to move in and out of system 2. Refocus on midlife marital and career issues 3. Beginning shift toward joint caring for older generation
5. Launching children and moving on	Accepting a multitude of exits from and entries into the family system	1. Renegotiation of marital system as a dyad 2. Development of adult-to-adult relationships between grown children and their parents 3. Realignment of relationships to include in-laws and grandchildren 4. Dealing with disabilities and death of parents (grandparents)
6. Families in later life	Accepting the shifting of generational roles	1. Maintaining own and/or couple functioning and interests in face of physiological decline; exploration of new familial and social role options 2. Support for a more central role of middle generation 3. Making room in the system for the wisdom and experience of the elderly, supporting the older generation without overfunctioning for them 4. Dealing with loss of spouse, siblings, and other peers and preparation for own death. Life review and integration.

From Carter and McGoldrick (1988), with permission.

difficulty committing themselves to relationships and form a pseudoinde-
pendent identity centered around work. Women may choose to define
themselves in relation to a male and postpone or forgo establishing an
independent identity.

Tasks

1. **Differentiation of self in relation to family of origin.** The young adult's
   shift toward adult status involves the development of a mutually
   respectful form of relating with his or her parents in which the young
   adult's parents can be appreciated for what they are. The young adult
   adjusts his view of his parents by neither making them into what they
   are not nor blaming them for what they could not be.
2. **Development of intimate peer relationships.** The emphasis is on the
   young adult's passing from an individual orientation to an interdependent orientation of self. There is no single mold of social experience for
   young adults to follow as they develop intimate relationships. During
   this task, young adults strive to bridge the gap between autonomy and
   attachment as they share themselves with others rather than using
   others as the source of self (Aylmer, 1988).
3. **Establishment of self in relation to work and financial independence.**
   In a young adult's early 20s, the "trying on" of various identities to test
   or refine career skills and interest is typical. The young adult who is
   committed to a career path or occupational choice by his or her mid- to
   late 20s is less vulnerable to self-doubt or decreased self-esteem than
   the young adult without direction, and generally functions produc-
   tively with little anxiety. Issues of competitiveness, expectations, and
   differences regarding work and financial goals require sorting through
   by the young adult and his or her family of origin.

Attachments

There are no right or wrong attachments for young adults in stage
one. Rather it is important for the nurse to draw forth from the family its
beliefs about attachment to each other and how it regards this attachment.
Some sample attachments for stage one are given in Figure 3–10. The first

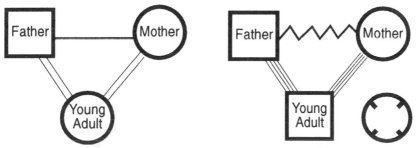

Figure 3–10. Sample attachments in stage 1.

diagram illustrates a young adult who is bonded equally with her father and mother. The second diagram illustrates a young adult who is more closely attached to each parent than the parents are to each other; the parents are negatively bonded. Of significance in the second diagram is that there was a death during the childhood of the young adult. It could be hypothesized that his difficulties in establishing his own identity are related to the family's hesitancy to come to grips with his deceased sister and the "empty nest."

Questions to Ask the Family. Who between your parents is most accepting of your career plans? How does he or she show this? What does your sister think of your parents' reaction to your career plans? If your father were more accepting of your desire to move into an independent living situation, how do you think your mother would react?

Stage Two: Marriage: The Joining of Families

Many couples believe that when they marry, it is just two individuals who are joining together. However, both spouses have grown up in families that have now become interconnected through marriage. Both spouses, although hopefully differentiated from their families of origin in an emotional, financial, and functional way, carry their whole family into the relationship. Marriage is a two-generational relationship with a minimum of three families coming together: his family of origin, her family of origin, and the new couple.

Tasks

1. **Establishment of couple identity.** The new couple must establish itself as an identifiable unit. This requires a negotiation of many issues that previously were defined on an individual level. These issues include such routine matters as eating and sleeping patterns, sexual contact, and use of space and time. The couple must decide about which traditions and rules to retain from each family and which ones they will develop for themselves.

2. **Realignment of relationships with extended families to include spouse.** A renegotiation of relationships with each spouse's family of origin has to take place to accommodate the new spouse. This can place no small stress on both the couple and each family of origin to open itself to new ways of being. Some couples deal with their parents by cutting off the relationship in a bid for independence. Other couples choose to handle this task of realignment by absorbing the new spouse into the enmeshed family of origin. The third common pattern involves a balance between some contact and some distance.

3. **Decisions about parenthood.** For most couples, experiencing happiness is highest at the beginning of the life cycle stage of marriage. Although a small but increasing number of married couples are deciding not to have children, most still plan on becoming parents. The

question of *when* to conceive is becoming increasingly complex, especially with the changing role of women, the widespread use of contraceptives, and the trend toward later marriages (Glick, 1989a). It has been found that couples who have evolved more competent marital structures prenatally are more likely to incorporate the child successfully into the family (Lewis, 1988a; Lewis, 1988b; Lewis, Owen, & Cox, 1988).

Attachments

A sample attachment for a couple in stage two is the development of close emotional ties between the spouses (Fig. 3–11). The first diagram illustrates how they do not have to break ties with their families of origin

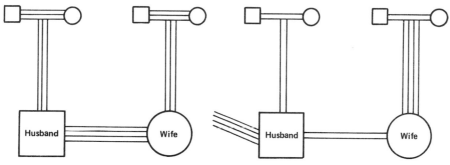

Figure 3–11. *Sample attachments in stage 2.*

but rather maintain ties with and adjust to them. A different type of attachment (illustrated in the second diagram) can occur if a couple does not align themselves together. The wife is more heavily bonded to her family of origin than she is to her husband. The husband is more tied to outside interests (e.g., work, friends) than to his wife.

Questions to Ask the Family. Which family was most in favor of your marriage? How did your siblings show that they supported your marriage? What did your spouse think of your parents' marital relationship? If you two as a couple were to model your marriage on your parents' marriage, what would you incorporate into your marriage?

Stage Three: Families with Young Children

During this stage, the adults now become caretakers to a younger generation. Issues about taking responsibility and dealing with the demands of dependent children are challenging for most families when financial resources are typically stretched and the parents are heavily involved in career development. The disposition of child-care responsibilities and household chores in dual-career households is a particular struggle. Schnittger and Bird (1990) found that men and women differ significantly in the coping strategies they use to deal with this issue. Women utilize cognitive restructuring, delegating, limiting avocational activities, and using social support significantly more often than do men.

As children progress in age, Schittger and Bird found that both men and women altered their use of coping strategies; for example, those with children under age 6 reported less use of delegating than those with an oldest child age 13 to 18.

Tasks

1. **Adjusting marital system to make space for child.** The couple must continue to meet each other's personal needs as well as meet their parental responsibilities. Both mothers and fathers are increasingly aware of the need for emotional integration of the child into the family. Children can be brought into a variety of environments: there is no space for them, there is space for them, or there is a vacuum that they are expected to fill. If the child has a handicap, there will be more stress on the couple as they adjust their expectations and deal with their emotional reactions.
2. **Joining in child-rearing, financial, and household tasks.** The couple must find a mutually satisfying way to deal with child-care responsibility and household chores that does not overburden one partner. The emotional as well as the financial cost of solutions to deal with child-care responsibilities must be addressed. Both mothers and fathers contribute to the child's development, but they do so in different ways. Evidence from both the home and laboratory setting indicate paternal physical and playful stimulation of the child complements maternal verbal interaction (Hanson & Bozett, 1986). Parents can either support or hinder their children's success in developing peer relationships and achieving at school. Middle-class families, responding to intense pressure from the school system, tend to stress the values of achievement and productivity, whereas some working-class families may respond to this pressure by feelings of alienation.
3. **Realignment of relationships with extended family to include parenting and grandparenting roles.** The couple must design and develop the new roles of father and mother in addition to the marital role rather than replacing it. Members of each family of origin also take on new roles, for example, grandpa or aunt. Frequently, grandparents who perhaps were opposed to the marriage in the beginning become very interested in the young children. For many older adults this is an especially gratifying time because it allows them to have intimacy without the responsibility required by parenting. It also permits them to develop a new type of adult-adult relationship with their children.

Attachments

Parents need to maintain a marital bond and continue personal adult-centered conversations in addition to child-centered conversations. Space for privacy and time spent together are important needs. Children

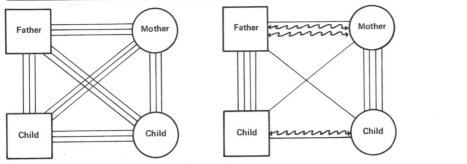

Figure 3–12. *Sample attachments in stage 3.*

require security and warm attachments to adults, as well as the opportunity to develop positive sibling relationships. In Figure 3–12, sample attachment diagrams are given. A competitive, negative relationship (illustrated by the wavy line) exists between the children and between the spouses in the second diagram. The mother is overbonded to the daughter, and the father is underinvolved with the daughter. The father is overattached to the son, and the mother is underinvolved with the son. This is an example of same-sex coalitions crossgenerationally.

Questions to Ask the Family. What percentage of your time do you spend taking care of your children? What percentage do you spend taking care of your marriage? Is this a comfortable balance for the two of you? What effect does this pattern have on your children? If your children thought that you should be closer, how might they tell you this?

Stage Four: Families with Adolescents

This period has often been characterized as one of intense upheaval and transition, in which biological, emotional, and sociocultural changes occur with great and ever-increasing rapidity.

Tasks

1. **Shift of parent-child relationships to permit adolescents to move in or out of system.** The family must move from the dependency relationship previously established with a young child to an increasingly independent relationship with the adolescent. Growing psychological independence is frequently not recognized due to continuing physical dependence. Conflict often surfaces when a teenager's independence threatens the family, who count on the teenager's dependency for their well-being. For example, teenagers may precipitate marital conflict when they question who makes the family rules about the car: Mom or Dad? Families frequently respond to an adolescent's request for increasing autonomy in two ways: (1) they abruptly define rigid rules and recreate an earlier stage of dependency or (2) they establish premature independence. In the second scenario, the family supports only independence

and ignores dependent needs. This may result in premature separation when the teenager is not really ready to be fully autonomous. The teenager may thus return home defeated.

2. **Refocus on midlife marital and career issues.** During this stage, parents are often struggling with what Erikson (1963) calls generativity, the need to be useful to another generation. The teenager's frequent questioning and conflict about values, lifestyles, career plans, and so forth can thrust the parents into an examination of their own marital and career issues.

3. **Beginning shift toward joint caring for older generation.** As parents are aging so too are the grandparents. Parents sometimes feel they are besieged on both sides: teenagers are asking for more freedom and grandparents are asking for more support.

Attachments

All family members continue to have their relationships within the family, or increasingly, the teenagers are more involved with their friends than with family members. The husband and wife need to reinvest in the marital relationship.

An example of an attachment pattern is illustrated in Figure 3–13. In

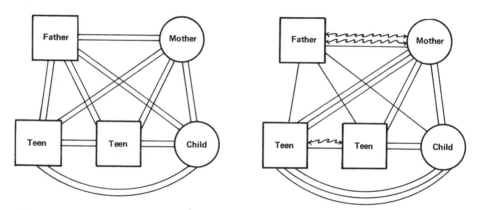

Figure 3–13. *Sample attachments in stage 4.*

the second diagram, the mother is overinvolved with the eldest son and has a negative relationship with the husband. The father tends to be minimally involved with all family members. There is conflict between the two sons.
Questions to Ask the Family. What privileges do your teenagers have now that they did not have when they were younger? *Ask the adolescents:* How do you think your parents will handle it when your younger sister wants to date? Will it be different from when you wanted to date?

Stage Five: Launching Children and Moving On

Growing numbers of middle-class North Americans whose children have grown up and left home assumed they would now have an empty nest. However, they are finding that their expectations are not being met. Rising housing costs and beginning pay rates that have not gone up as fast as those of more experienced workers have been singled out as the natural causes of this trend. Recent ideas suggest a different explanation: young North Americans are having difficulty growing up and are unwilling to go out on their own and settle for less affluence than their parents. In a *New York Times* article, "Parenthood II: The nest won't stay empty" (1989), it was reported that "18 million single adults 18–34 years (in the United States) were living with parents, an increase of about one-third since 1974. The trend is more than a trickle" (p. 1).

Tasks

1. **Renegotiation of marital system as a dyad.** There is frequently a thrust to alter some of the basic tenets of the marital relationship. This is especially true if both partners are working and the children have left home. The couple bond can take on a more prominent position. The balance between dependency, independency, and interdependency has to be reexamined.
2. **Development of adult-to-adult relationships between grown children and their parents.** The family of origin must relinquish the primary roles of parent and child. They must adapt to the new roles of parent and separate adult. This involves renegotiation of emotional and financial commitments. There is decreased investment in caretaking activities by the parents and increased investment in physical separation and independent living by the young adult. The key emotional process during this stage is for family members to deal with a multitude of exits from and entries into the family system.
3. **Realignment of relationships to include in-laws and grown children.** The parents adjust family ties and expectations to include their child's spouse or partner. Although earlier studies have viewed this phase as a lonely, sad time, especially for women, Lupri and Frideres (1981) have noted an increase in marital satisfaction during the postparental stage.
4. **Dealing with disabilities and death of grandparents.** Many families regard the disability or death of an elderly parent as a natural occurrence. If however, there is unfinished business between the couple and the elderly parents, this may have serious repercussions, not only for the children but also for the new third generation. The type of disability afflicting the seniors will determine its effects on the immediate family. For example, Pallett (1990) points out that caregivers who do not understand Alzheimer's dementia and its effects on cognitive function and behavior often attempt to deal with inappropriate or disruptive behavior in ineffective and counterproductive ways. They thus inadvertently intensify their own stress.

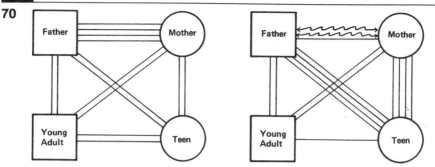

Figure 3–14. *Sample attachments in stage 5.*

Attachments

Each family member continues to have outside interests and establishes new roles appropriate to this stage. Sample attachment patterns are illustrated in Figure 3–14. A problem may arise when both husband and wife hold on to their last child. They may avoid conflict by allowing the eldest child to leave home but then focus on the next one.

Questions to Ask the Family. How did your parents help you to leave home? What is the difference between how you left home and how your children are leaving home? Will your parents get along better, worse, or the same with each other once you have left home? Who, between your mom and dad, will miss the children the most? As you see your child moving on with a new relationship, what would you like your child to do differently than you did? If your parents are still alive, are there any issues you would like to discuss with them?

Stage Six: Families in Later Life

This stage begins with retirement and lasts until the death of both spouses. Potentially, it can last 20 to 25 years for many couples. The key emotional process in this stage is to accept the shift of generational roles.

Tasks

1. **Maintaining own and/or couple functioning and interest in the face of physiological decline: exploration of new familial and social role options.** Marital relationships continue to be important, and marital satisfaction contributes to both the morale and ongoing activity of both spouses. Bishop, Epstein, Baldwin, Miller, and Keitner (1988) found that the husband's morale is most strongly associated with health, socioeconomic status, and income, and to a lesser extent, with family functioning. The wife's morale is most strongly associated with family functioning, and to a lesser extent, with health and socioeconomic status.

   As the older couple find themselves in new roles of grandparents and mother-in-law and father-in-law, they must adjust to their children's spouses and open space for the new grandchildren. Difficulty in making the status changes required can be reflected in an older family member refusing to relinquish some of his or her power: for example, refusing to turn over a company or making plans for succession in a family business. The shift in status between the senior family members and the middle-aged family members is a reciprocal one. Difficulties may occur in several ways: if older adults give up and become totally dependent on the next generation, if the next generation does not accept the seniors' diminishing powers and treats them as totally competent, or if the next generation sees only the seniors' frailties and treats them as totally incompetent.

2. **Making room in the system for the wisdom and experience of the seniors.** The task of supporting the older generation without overfunctioning for them is particularly salient as people are living longer. The vast majority of adults over 65 do not live alone but rather with other family members, and less than 5 percent live in institutions. It is not uncommon to have a 90-year-old parent being cared for by her 70-year-old daughter, with both of them living in close proximity to a 50-year-old son/grandson. Giordano (1988) comments that the parents of the baby boomers will be the next generation of "young-old." He believes they will be highly motivated to participate in self-help groups and will be interested in improving their quality of life through counseling, health activities, and education. "They will not accept the aging myths of the past: they will not just expect a better quality of life—they will help command society and, in so doing, control their destiny" (p. 414).

3. **Dealing with loss of spouse, siblings, and other peers and preparation for death.** This is a time for life review and taking care of unfinished business with family as well as with business and social contacts. Many people find it helpful to discuss their life, review it, and enjoy the opportunity of passing this information along to succeeding generations.

Attachments

The couple reinvest and modify the marital relationship based on the level of functioning of both partners. There is an appropriate interdependence with the next generation. This concept of interdependence is particularly important for nurses to understand in working with families with adult daughters and their parents. Middle-class older men and women seem equally likely to aid and support their children, especially daughters. Frequency of contact, however, tends to be higher with daughters than with sons. Thus, the possibility of strong intergenerational attachments between a daughter and her parents exist. In the attachment pattern illustrated in Figure 3–15, the couple project their conflicts onto the extended family. This causes difficulty for the succeeding generations. *Questions to Ask the Family.* When you look back over your life, what

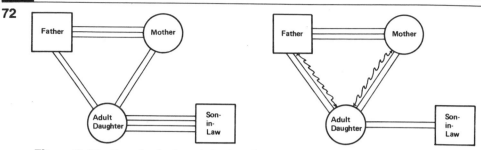

Figure 3–15. *Sample attachments in stage 6.*

aspects have you enjoyed the most? What has given you the most happiness? About what aspects do you feel the most regret? What would you hope that your children would do differently than you did? Similarly to what you did?

THE DIVORCE AND POSTDIVORCE FAMILY LIFE CYCLE

The largest variation from the middle-class North American family life cycle is the life cycle of those families who go through divorce and postdivorce. Glick (1989a) states that "one of the main reasons why the original model for the family life cycle has become outmoded is the now familiar upsurge in divorce and decline in remarriage" (p. 125). The divorce rate was more than twice as high in 1987 as in 1960. Whether the divorce rate will climb, level off, or decline is a matter of speculation that can be backed up by various theories. There may be pressure for divorce to decline somewhat because of the possibility of stable economic conditions and the AIDS epidemic. "The number of divorced mothers increased in the United States at an average rate of 9% a year in the 1970's but the census bureau reports that it has increased by only 1.6% annually since 1980" (Suro, 1991, p. 2).

Most divorces occur early in marriage. "The median duration of all marriages that ended in divorce in 1988 was 7.1 years, the highest in 20 years. First marriages lasted approximately 2 years longer before divorce than second marriages, which in turn lasted 2 years longer than third or subsequent marriages" (Divorce rate drops, 1991, p. 16). In the United States the divorce rate dropped in 1988 for the third straight year. Glick (1989a) found that single parents constituted 11 percent of all families in the United States in 1988, with about 1 out of every 7 of these families being maintained by the father, as compared with 1 out of every 10 in 1960.

Families experiencing divorce are often under enormous pressure. Hill (1986) comments that single-parent families must accomplish most of the same developmental tasks as two-parent families, but without all the resources. This places extra burdens on the remaining family members, who must compensate with increased effort to accomplish family tasks such as physical maintenance, social control, and tension management.

Quinn and Allen (1989) indicated from their study of 30 employed single parents that there were challenges in managing shortages of time, money, and energy. These parents voiced serious concerns about failure to meet perceived family and societal expectations for living "in a normal family" with two parents. "The women feel they must display behaviors which are contradictory to those they assumed they should exhibit if they were to remarry" (p. 390). They perceived ongoing pressure from family, friends, and church to marry again to give their children a "normal" family. The women reported being caught in a double bind, trying to demonstrate behaviors that might net them a new husband while trying to use seemingly opposing behaviors that allowed them to successfully manage their lives. We encourage nurses working with single-parent families to explore the parent's feelings about opposing expectations. This is a way of helping the women to plan their responses to various paradoxical situations. In our clinical supervision with nurses, we encourage focusing on the siblings, a subsystem that generally remains intact during the process of family reorganization. Schibuk (1989) reasons that sibling therapy can be effective, as children are the "unit of continuity" (p. 226).

Because divorce may occur at any stage of the family life cycle, it has a different impact on family functioning depending on its timing. The marital breakdown may be sudden or it may be long and drawn out. In either case, emotional work is required so that the family may deal with the shifts, gains, and losses in family membership. The phases involved in divorce and postdivorce are depicted in Table 3–2. Carter and McGoldrick (1988) have found a clinical usefulness in the distinctions made between the three columns given in the tables. Column 1 lists the phase. Column 2 gives the prerequisite attitudes that will assist family members to make the transition and come through the developmental issues listed in column 3 en route to the next phase. We believe that clinical work directed at column 3 will not succeed if the family is having difficulty dealing with the issues in column 2.

Questions to Ask the Family. How do you explain to yourself the reasons for your divorce? Who initiated the idea of divorce? Who left whom? Who was most supportive of developing viable arrangements for *everyone* in the family? How was your spouse's willingness to continue a cooperative coparental relationship shown? How did you respond to this? As you resolved your attachment to your spouse, what changes did you notice in your children? What would your in-laws say about how you have fostered your children's relationship with them? What would your children say? What methods have you found most successful in resolving conflicting issues with your ex-spouse? What advice would you give to other divorced parents on how to resolve conflictual issues with their ex-partners? How have your children helped you and your ex-spouse to maintain a supportive environment for them?

TABLE 3–2 STAGES OF DIVORCE FAMILY LIFE CYCLE

Phase	Emotional Process of Transition, Prerequisite Attitude	Developmental Issues
Divorce		
1. Deciding to divorce	Accepting inability to resolve marital tensions sufficiently to continue relationship	Accepting one's own part in the failure of the marriage
2. Planning the break-up of the system	Supporting viable arrangements for all parts of the system	a. Working cooperatively on problems of custody, visitation, and finances b. Dealing with extended family about the divorce
3. Separation	a. Being willing to continue cooperative coparental relationship and joint financial support of children b. Working on resolution of attachment to spouse	a. Mourning loss of nuclear family b. Restructuring marital and parent-child relationships and finances; adaptation to living apart c. Realigning relationships with extended family; staying connected with spouse's extended family
4. Divorce	More work on emotional divorce: overcoming hurt, anger, guilt, and so forth	a. Retrieving hopes, dreams, and expectations from the marriage
Postdivorce		
1. Single-parent (custodial household or primary residence)	Being willing to maintain financial responsibilities, continue parental contact with ex-spouse, and support contact of children with ex-spouse and his or her family	a. Making flexible visitation arrangements with ex-spouse and his or her family b. Rebuilding own financial resources c. Rebuilding own social network
2. Single-parent (non-custodial)	Being willing to maintain parental contact with ex-spouse and support custodial parent's relationship with children	a. Finding ways to continue effective parenting relationship with children b. Maintaining financial responsibilities to ex-spouse and children c. Rebuilding own social network

Adapted from Carter and McGoldrick (1988).

REMARRIED FAMILY LIFE CYCLE

The rise of the remarried and the stepfamily in North America in the recent decade has been striking. Between two thirds and three fourths of those who divorce eventually remarry. Glick (1989a) states that he sees "a preference for marriage in the observation that nine-tenths of young Americans are likely to marry; that close to one-half of the first marriages are likely to remain intact, despite the many options available to those involved; and that between two-thirds and three-fourths of those who divorce will eventually remarry" (p. 129). Glick (1989a) reports an expected 72 percent of recently divorced women remarry. The level is higher (81 percent) for divorced women with no children, about the same (73 percent) for those with one or two children, and considerably lower (57 percent) for those with three or more children.

Glick (1989b) discusses the differences between a remarried family and a stepfamily with the latter being a "family remarried with a child under 18 years of age who is the biological child of one of the parents and was born before the remarriage occurred" (p. 24). In 1987, Glick estimates there were 11 million remarried families and 4.3 million stepfamilies in the United States. He states that "21.3% of married couples/families are remarried families and 8.3% of all married couples/families are stepfamilies" (p. 25).

Pill (1990) states that the redivorce rate for remarried couples is even higher than the divorce rate following first marriages. The high rate of redivorce within the first 5 years of remarriage suggests that these early years are a challenging period. Pill (1990) studied 29 nonclincal stepfamilies with custodial adolescent stepchildren and examined cohesion and adaptability. He found that they were in the process of revising their basic assumptions about family life and developing a stepfamily identity. The stepfamilies reported low to moderate levels of cohesion and moderate to high levels of adaptability, both of which were associated with stepfamily but not marital satisfaction. Stepfamily cohesion was lower than that of nuclear families, whereas adaptability was higher in the same life cycle stage.

The family emotional process at the transition to remarriage consists of struggling with fears about investment in new relationships: one's own fears, the new spouse's fears, and the fears of the children (of either or both spouses). It also consists of dealing with hostile or upset reactions of the children, the extended families, and ex-spouse. There is a need to address the ambiguity of the new family organization, including roles and relationships. Oftentimes there is an increased arousal of parental guilt and concerns about the children, and there may be a positive or negative rearousal of the old attachment to the ex-spouse (Carter & McGoldrick, 1988). In Table 3–3 Carter and McGoldrick (1988) have given a developmental outline for stepfamily formation.

Ahrons and Rodgers (1987) have advocated for models of healthy,

TABLE 3–3 REMARRIED FAMILY FORMATION: A DEVELOPMENTAL OUTLINE

Steps	Prerequisite Attitude	Developmental Issues
1. Entering the new relationship	Recovery from loss of first marriage (adequate "emotional divorce")	Recommiting to marriage and to forming a family with readiness to deal with the complexity and ambiguity
2. Conceptualizing and planning the new marriage and family	Accepting one's own fears and those of new spouse and children about remarriage and forming a stepfamily Accepting need for time and patience for adjustment to complexity and ambiguity of: 1. Multiple new roles 2. Boundaries: space, time, membership, authority 3. Affective issues: guilt, loyalty conflicts, desire for mutuality, unresolvable past hurts	a. Working on openness in the new relationships to avoid pseudomutuality b. Planning for maintenance of cooperative financial and coparental relationships with ex-spouses c. Planning to help children deal with fears, loyalty conflicts, and membership in two systems d. Realigning relationships with extended family to include new spouse and children e. Planning maintenance of connections for children with extended family of ex-spouse(s)
3. Remarriage and reconstitution of family	Final resolution of attachment to previous spouse and ideal of "intact" family Accepting a different model of family with permeable boundaries	a. Restructuring family boundaries to allow for inclusion of new spouse-stepparent b. Realignment of relationships and financial arrangements throughout subsystems to permit interweaving of several systems c. Making room for relationships of all children with biological (noncustodial) parents, grandparents, and other extended family d. Sharing memories and histories to enhance stepfamily integration

From Carter and McGoldrick (1988), with permission.

well-functioning binuclear families. Having been angered by a predominant emphasis on pathology in the divorce literature, Ahrons began to study what she calls binuclear families. This term does not refer only to joint custody families or to families in which the relationship between ex-spouses is friendly but rather indicates a different familial structure, without inferring anything about the nature or quality of the ex-spouses' relationship. Ahrons and Rodgers, who worked with 98 divorced couples over a 5-year period, produced some interesting relationship types, including "perfect pals," a small group of divorced spouses whose previous marriage had not overshadowed their longstanding friendship. The "cooperative colleagues" were a considerably larger and typical group found by Ahrons and Rodgers. Although not good friends, they worked well together on issues concerning their children. The third group were the "angry associates," and the fourth group were "fiery foes," who felt nothing but fury for their ex-spouses. Ahrons and Rodgers termed the fifth group "dissolved duos," who after the separation or divorce discontinued any contact with each other.

We encourage nurses working with divorced and remarried families to bring their patients/clients research knowledge of what works or does not work to foster continuing family relationships. Nurses should be cautioned, however, that there are seldom simple answers to complex problems. For example, Healy, Malley, and Stewart (1990) found that predictors such as child's age, gender, frequency and regularity of father-child visitation, father-child closeness, and parental legal conflict on the child's self-esteem were found to have different implications for different groups of 6- to 12-year-old children and for children in different situations. Their findings "suggest the futility of seeking simple answers to whether ongoing contact with fathers following divorce is beneficial or detrimental for children" (p. 531).

Questions to Ask the Family. What were the differences between you and your spouse in how you each successfully recovered from your first marriage? What most helped each of you deal with your own fears about remarriage? About forming a stepfamily? How did your spouse invite your children to adjust to him or her? What do your children think was the most useful thing you did in helping them deal with loyalty conflicts. What advice do you have for other stepfamilies on how to create a new family? What are you most proud of in how you have helped your stepfamily successfully make the transition from what they were before to what they are now?

COMPARISON OF PROFESSIONAL AND LOW-INCOME FAMILY LIFE CYCLE STAGES

The family life cycle of the poor frequently does not match the middle-class paradigm so often used to conceptualize their situations. Hines (1988) suggests that the family life cycle of the poor is actually three phases: the unattached young adult (perhaps younger than 12 years old) who is virtually unaccountable to any adults, families with children—a phase occupying most of the life span and including three- and four-generational households, and the final phase of the grandmother who is still involved in central childrearing in her senior years. It has been estimated that 9.7 percent of American children lived in a household headed by someone other than a parent in 1990, up from 6.7 percent in 1970 (Gross, 1992). We

TABLE 3–4 COMPARISON OF FAMILY LIFE CYCLE STAGES

Age	Professional Families	Low-Income Families
12–17	a. Prevent pregnancy b. Graduate from high school c. Parents continue support while permitting child to achieve greater independence	a. First pregnancy b. Attempt to graduate from high school c. Parent attempts strict control before pregnancy. After pregnancy, relaxation of controls and continued support of new mother and infant
18–21	a. Prevent pregnancy b. Leave parental household for college c. Adapt to parent-child separation	a. Second pregnancy b. No further education c. Young mother acquires adult status in parental household
22–25	a. Prevent pregnancy b. Develop professional identity in graduate school c. Maintain separation from parental household. Begin living in serious relationship	a. Third pregnancy b. Marriage: leave parental household to establish stepfamily c. Maintain connection with kinship network
26–30	a. Prevent pregnancy b. Marriage: develop nuclear couple as separate from parents c. Intense work involvement as career begins	a. Separate from husband b. Mother becomes head of own household within kinship network
31–35	a. First pregnancy b. Renew contact with parents as grandparents c. Differentiate career and child-rearing roles between husband and wife	a. First grandchild b. Mother becomes grandmother and cares for daughter and infant

From Fulmer (1988), with permission.

encourage nurses to consider the effects of ethnicity and religion, socioeconomic status, race, and environment on how, when, and what way a family makes its own transitions in its own life cycle.

Fulmer (1988) has suggested one comparison of the life cycle stages of professional and low-income families. His comparisons are outlined in Table 3–4. We encourage nurses to consider the great variability between various types of families as well as within types of families.

ADOPTIVE FAMILY LIFE CYCLE

In adoption, the family boundaries of all those involved are expanded. Reitz and Watson (1992) define adoption as

A means of providing some children with security and meeting their developmental needs by legally transferring ongoing parental responsibilities from their birth parents to their adoptive parents; recognizing that in so doing we have created a new kinship network that forever links those two families together through the child, who is shared by both. (p. 11)

We agree with this definition. As in marriage, the new legal status of the adoptive family does not automatically sever the psychological ties to the earlier family. Rather, the family boundaries are expanded and realigned.

We believe that nurses should be aware of the trends and special circumstances in forming adoptive families. For example, most agencies offer adoption service along a continuum of openness. There also can be divorced, single-parent, married, or remarried adoptive families. Reitz and Watson (1992) also have discussed adoptions within extended families as well as families with various forms of open dual parentage.

The adoption process, including the decision, application, and final adoption, can be a stressful as well as a joyful period for many couples. During the preschool developmental phase, the family must acknowledge the adoption as a fact of family life. The question of the permanency of the relationship sometimes arises from both the child and the parents. Hajal and Rosenberg (1991) have developed some hypotheses to explain the overrepresentation of adopted children (particularly those between 11 and 16) in the mental health outpatient system:

1. Genetic, heredity factors
2. Deficiencies in prenatal and perinatal care
3. Adverse circumstances of adoption, including multiple disruptions in early life
4. Conditions in the adoptive home, including preexisting family problems
5. Temperamental differences between the adoptee and the adoptive parents or family
6. Fantasy system and communication regarding adoption, including parental attitudes about adoption
7. Difficulties establishing a firm sense of identity during adolescence
8. Greater age difference than usual between parents and adoptees

We believe it is important for nurses to recognize adoptive families' strengths and resources as they deal with these challenging issues. During the adolescent stage of family development, the major task is to increase flexibility of family boundaries. In adoptive families, altercations may give rise to threats of desertion or rejection. During the young adult or launching phase, the young adult "adopts" the parents in a recontracting phase according to Hajal and Rosenberg (1991). As the adopted child proceeds to develop his or her own family of procreation, the integration of the adoptee's biological progeny can be a developmental challenge for everyone. Adoptive parents may be delighted with the psychological and social continuity. Simultaneously, they may mourn the loss of biological grandchildren and the pain of genealogical discontinuity. For the adoptee, reproduction includes both the thrill of a biological relationship and maybe some fears of the unknowns in their own genetic history.

In this CFAM developmental category, we have presented five sample types of family life cycles. Nursing has only begun to recognize the special characteristics of other family forms, such as gay male and lesbian couples. We encourage nurses to broaden their perspectives when interacting with various family forms. It is very difficult and not clinically useful to depict *the* family form of the 1990s. What we do know is that there is great variety: the poor and homeless family, lesbian or gay male couple, single parent, adopted child with parent, stepfamily, divorced family, separated family, nuclear family, and extended family. There will also be children living in households not headed by a parent (Gross, 1992).

FUNCTIONAL ASSESSMENT

The family functional assessment is concerned with details of how individuals *actually* behave in relation to one another. It is the here-and-now aspect of a family's life, which is observed and that the family presents. There are two basic aspects to family functioning: instrumental and expressive (Parsons & Bales, 1956). Each will be dealt with separately.

INSTRUMENTAL FUNCTIONING

The instrumental aspect of family functioning refers to the routine activities of daily living, such as eating, sleeping, preparing meals, giving injections, changing dressings, and so forth. For families with health problems, this is a particularly important area. The instrumental activities of daily life are generally more numerous, more frequent, and take on a greater significance because of a family member's illness. A quadriplegic, for example, requires assistance with almost every instrumental task. If a baby is attached to an apnea monitor, the parents almost always alter the manner in which they take care of instrumental tasks. One parent, for example, will only leave the apartment to do a load of wash if the other parent is sufficiently awake to attend to the infant. If a senior family member is unable to distinguish what medication to take at a specific time, other family members often alter their daily routines to telephone or drop in on the senior.

EXPRESSIVE FUNCTIONING

The expressive aspect refers to nine categories:

1. Emotional communication
2. Verbal communication
3. Nonverbal communication
4. Circular communication
5. Problem-solving
6. Roles
7. Influence
8. Beliefs
9. Alliances/coalitions

These nine subcategories are derived in part from the Family Categories Schema first developed by Epstein, Sigal, and Rakoff (1968) and later published by Epstein, Bishop, and Levin (1978). These categories were expanded by Tomm in 1977 and later published by Tomm and Sanders (1983). Earlier work (Westley & Epstein, 1969) had suggested that several of these categories distinguished emotionally healthy families from those that were experiencing more than the usual emotional distress. We have expanded on these works and now include nonverbal and circular communication as well as beliefs (see Table 8–3).

Before discussing each subcategory, we would like to point out that most families have to deal with a combination of instrumental and expressive issues. For example, an older woman has a burn. The instrumental issues revolve around dressing changes and an exercise program. The expressive or affective issues might center on roles or problem-solving. The family might be considering the following questions:

Whose role is it to change Gram's dressing?
Are women better "nurses" than men?
Whose turn is it to call the physical therapist?
Why is it that Milton never gets involved in Gram's care?
How can we get Milton to drive Gram to see the doctor?

If a family is not coping well with instrumental issues, then expressive issues almost always exist. However, a family can deal well with instrumental issues and still have expressive or emotional difficulties. It is therefore useful for the nurse to delineate the instrumental from the expressive issues. Both need to be explored in a thorough family assessment.

Although both past behaviors and future goals are taken into consideration in the functional assessment, the primary focus is on the here-and-now. It is helpful to identify a family's strengths and limitations in each of the following subcategories. We find it helpful to remember that family assessment is the evaluation of a family system. Patterns of interaction are the main thrust of the functional assessment category. Families are obviously composed of individuals, but the focus of a family assessment is less on the individual and more on the interaction *among* all of the individuals within the family. Thus, the family is viewed as a system of interacting members. In conducting this part of the family assessment, the nurse operates under the assumption that individuals are best understood within their immediate social context. The nurse conceives of the individual as defining and being defined by that context. The individual's relationships with family members and other meaningful members of the larger social environment are thus very important.

By interviewing family members together, the nurse can observe how they spontaneously interact and influence each other. Furthermore, the nurse can ask questions about the impact family members have on one another and on the health problem. Reciprocally, the nurse can enquire about the impact of the health problem on the family. If the nurse thinks "interactionally" rather than "individually," then each individual family member's behavior will not be seen in isolation but rather will be understood in context.

Emotional Communication

This subcategory refers to the range and types of emotions or feelings that are expressed or shown or both. Families generally express a wide spectrum of feelings from happiness to sadness to anger, whereas families with difficulties often have quite rigid patterns within a narrow range of emotional expression. For example, some families experiencing difficulties almost always argue and rarely show affection. In other families, parents may express anger but children may not, or the family may have no difficulty with women expressing tenderness but men are not permitted to do this.

Questions to Ask the Family. Who in the family tends to start conversations about feelings? How can you tell when your dad is feeling happy? Angry? Sad? How about your mom? What effect does your anger have on your son? What does your mom do when your dad is angry? If your grandmother were to express sadness to your parents, how do you think your parents would react?

Verbal Communication

This subcategory focuses primarily on the relationship expressed by the verbal content, and only secondarily on that expressed by the semantic content, of a communication. That is, the focus is on the meaning of the words in terms of the relationship.

Direct communication implies that the message is sent to the intended target. An elderly woman may be upset with what her husband is saying, but corrects her grandson's inconsequential fidgeting with the comment, "Stop doing that to me." This could represent a displaced message, whereas the same statement directed at her husband would be considered direct.

Clear versus masked is another way of looking at verbal communication. It refers to the lack of distortion in the message. A father's statement to his child, "Children who cry when they get needles are babies" may be masked criticism if the child is fighting back tears at the time of his injection.

Questions to Ask the Family. Who among your family members is the most clear and direct when communicating verbally? When you are clear with your young adult son that he has to pay rent to you, what effect does that have on him? When your teenagers talk directly to each other about the use of condoms, what do you notice? If your adolescents were to talk more with you and your husband about safe sex, what do you think his reaction might be?

Nonverbal Communication

This subcategory focuses on the various nonverbal and paraverbal messages that family members communicate. Nonverbal messages include body position, eye contact, touch, gestures, and so forth. The proximity or distance between family members is also an important nonverbal communication. Paraverbals include tonality, guttural sounds, crying, stammering, and so forth.

Nurses should attend to the sequence of nonverbal messages as well as to their timing. For example, when an older man starts to talk about his terminal illness and his adult daughter turns her head and casts her tear-filled eyes to the floor, then the nurse can infer that the daughter is sad about her father's impending death. Her sequence of nonverbal behavior is congruent with sadness and the topic of conversation. It is not necessarily, however, the most supportive sequence for her father.

Questions to Ask the Family. Who in your family shows the most distress when your father is drinking? How does Sheldon show it? What does your mother do when your father is drinking? When your brother turns his head and stares out the window as your father is talking, what effect does it have on you? If your dad were to stop talking at the same time as your mother, what do you think she would feel like saying to him?

Circular Communication

This subcategory refers to the reciprocal communication between persons (Watzlawick, Beavin, & Jackson, 1967). There is a pattern to most relationship issues. For example, a common circular pattern occurs when the wife feels angry and criticizes her husband; the husband feels angry and he avoids the issues and her. The more he avoids, the more angry she becomes. The wife tends to see the problem only as her husband's, whereas the husband identifies the wife's criticism as the only problem. The circularity of this pattern is the most important aspect in understanding interaction in dyads. Each person influences the behavior of the other. More information about this is available in Chapter 2.

These circular communication patterns can also be adaptive. For example, an older parent feels competent and negotiates well with the landlord; the adult son feels proud and praises his parent. The more reinforcement the adult son gives, the more confident and self-assured the senior feels. This pattern is diagrammed in Figure 3–16.

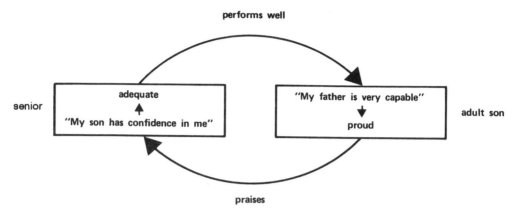

Figure 3–16. *Adaptive circular pattern diagram.*

Circular pattern diagrams (CPDs) concretize and simplify repetitive sequences noted in a relationship. This method of diagramming interaction patterns was first developed by Tomm (1980). The simplest CPD includes two behaviors and two inferences of meaning. The inferences used are cognitive or affective or both. Inferences about cognition refer to ideas, concepts, or beliefs, whereas inferences about affect refer to emotional states. Affect or cognition, or both, propel the behavior. Figure 3–17 illustrates the relationship between these elements.

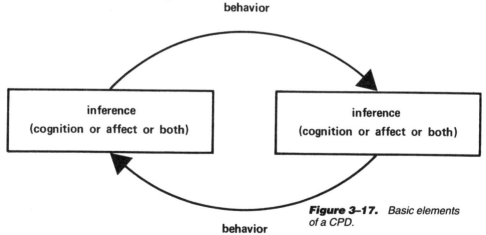

Figure 3–17. *Basic elements of a CPD.*

"The inference is entered inside the enclosure and represents some internal process (what is going on inside each interactant). The connecting arrows represent information conveyed from each person to the other through behavior. The circular linkage implies an interaction pattern that is repetitive, stable, and self-regulatory" (Tomm, 1980, p. 8). An example

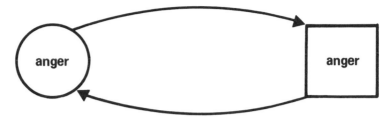

blames/threatens

Figure 3–18. *CPD of a circular argument.*

blames/threatens

of a circular argument is illustrated in Figure 3–18. Each party blames and threatens the other.

A supportive relationship is illustrated in Figure 3–19. The husband trusts his wife and reveals his needs and fears. She is concerned and in turn sustains and supports him. This leads him to trust her more, and the relationship progresses.

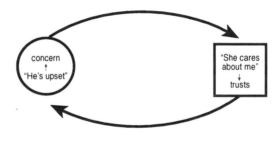

SUSTAINS/SUPPORTS

Figure 3–19. *CPD of a supportive relationship.*

EXPRESSES HIS NEEDS/FEARS

Questions to Ask the Family

Nurse: You say your wife always criticizes you. (Nurse conceptualizes Fig. 3–20). What do you do then? (Trying to fill in the husband's behavior in Fig. 3–21.)

Husband: I don't like to discuss things. I avoid conflict. I leave. I go in the other room. What else can I do? She's always telling me what I did wrong.

Nurse: So she expresses her needs and you leave. How do you think that makes her feel? (Trying to fill in the inferred emotion in the wife's circle in Fig. 3–22.)

Wife: I'll tell you. I get annoyed. I feel ignored, rejected.

Nurse: So you're annoyed when he leaves and ignores you. And then you become more critical. Is that right?

Wife: Well I don't really criticize, I just. . . .

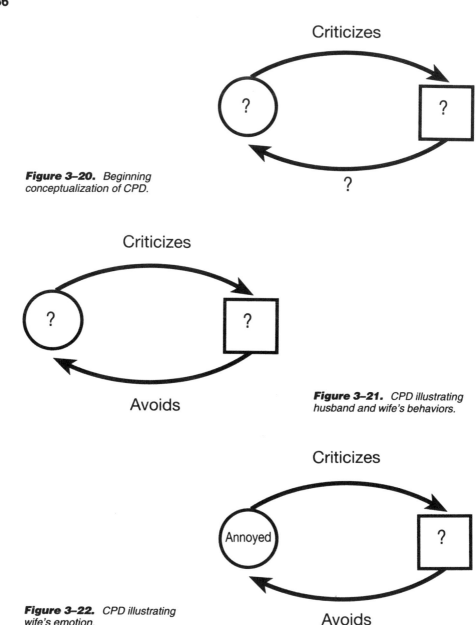

Figure 3–20. *Beginning conceptualization of CPD.*

Figure 3–21. *CPD illustrating husband and wife's behaviors.*

Figure 3–22. *CPD illustrating wife's emotion.*

Husband:	Yeah, you got it, nurse.
Nurse:	So, when you try and express your concerns, how do you think it makes him feel? (Trying to fill in the inference in the square in Fig. 3–22.)

Wife: I don't know.

Nurse: If he thinks you're lecturing, and he avoids the issues by leaving the room, what effect do you think your talking might be having on him?

Wife: Well, I suppose he could be feeling frustrated. He sulks.

Nurse: So the pattern seems to be that no matter who starts it, the circle completes itself: Sometimes you're annoyed and you criticize. Your husband feels frustrated and he ignores you. He sulks in the garage. Other times he avoids issues for whatever reason and this invites your frustration and criticism. (Explaining Fig. 3–23.)

Wife: It's a vicious circle.

Husband: I don't want it to go on this way any more. We both get too upset.

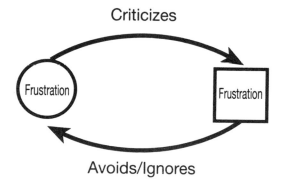

Figure 3–23. Nurse's conceptualization of this couple's communication pattern.

Problem-Solving

This subcategory refers to the family's ability to solve its own problems effectively. Who identifies the problems is important. Is it characteristically someone from outside the family or from inside the family?

Once the problems are identified by someone, are they mainly instrumental (routine, day-to-day logistics) or are they emotional problems? Families get into difficulties when they identify an emotional problem as an instrumental one. For example, a mother who states that she cannot get her child who has phenylketonuria (PKU) to keep to the diet is really discussing an emotional issue rather than an instrumental one. She has difficulty influencing her child.

What are the family's solution patterns? Many close-knit, extended families rely on relatives for assistance in time of need. Others tend to seek help from professionals. Knowing a family's usual solution style can give the nurse insight into why this family may be stuck at this particular time with this particular issue. For example, older parents move to a retirement community. The wife breaks her hip. The husband is used to being self-reliant or, in a pinch, depending on his middle-aged daughter. The older couple know few people in their new community. The husband is reluctant to accept help from the visiting nurse. He states he can manage all his wife's care despite the fact that he is losing weight and getting insufficient rest himself. The husband's solution pattern will be in conflict with that of the nurse.

Knowledge of whether or not a family evaluates the cost of its solutions can be helpful to the nurse. For example, a 68-year-old grandmother told Louise, the nurse, "I can't afford to let myself cry about the death of my son's infant. I have to go on for the sake of my other children." Louise was able to evaluate, with the grandmother, the cost of her solution pattern. Neither the grandmother nor the son discussed the infant's death with each other. The grandchildren's questions about "how come the baby didn't come home from the hospital" were left unanswered. There was considerable tension, and the son was particularly overprotective with the 4-year-old boy (the only surviving male child). By gently exploring the cost of the solution (tension and overprotection), the nurse was able to suggest other solution patterns (e.g., shared grieving).

Questions to Ask the Family. Who first noticed the problem? Are you the one who usually notices such things? What most helped you to take the first step toward eliminating the violence pattern? What effect did it have when you took steps to stop the cycle of violence in your family? How did the relationship between your son and and your husband change when the violence stopped? If a violent episode were to occur again, how do you think you and your daughter would deal with it?

Roles

This subcategory refers to the established patterns of behavior for family members. A role is consistent behavior in a particular situation. Roles, however, are not static but rather are developed through an individual's interactions with others. Roles are thus influenced by others' sanctions and norms. McGoldrick (1988b) writes that the idea that women have a life cycle apart from their roles as wife and mother is a relatively recent one and still is not widely accepted in our culture. The expectation for women has been that they would take care of the needs of others, first men, then children, then the older generation.

Parks and Pilisuk (1991) examined the psychological cost of providing care for a parent with Alzheimer's disease and found that anxiety, depression, guilt, and resentment were evident. That women dominated their sample of adult caregivers of a parent with Alzheimer's disease reflects an American pattern. The gender differences clearly profile women's more frequent, intensive, affective involvement with the caregiver role.

Women's roles are changing in recent years and are now less defined by the men in their lives. The birth rate has fallen below replacement levels, and many more women are concentrating on jobs and education. Nevertheless, women still make on average less than men do for the same job. Research has shown that a husband's income is negatively related to role sharing and the wife's education is positively related to role sharing (Ericksen, Yancey, & Ericksen, 1979).

Although role change is increasingly prevalent for both men and women in today's society, what is important for nurses to assess is how the family members cope with their roles. Is there role conflict or cooperation? Can the members cope with their roles? Are roles determined solely by age, rank order, or gender? Are there additional criteria? Are the women in the family more involved with a wider network of people for whom they feel responsible? Do the men hear less than the women in the family about stress in their family network?

Formal roles are those for which the community has broadly agreed on a norm. Examples include the roles of mother, husband, and friend. Informal roles refer to the established patterns of behavior that are idiosyncratic to particular individuals in certain settings. Examples include the roles of "softy," "angel," and "scapegoat." These serve a specific function in a particular family. If Dad is the "softy," then most likely Mom is the "heavy." If Giffy is the "good daughter," then probably David is the "black sheep." The roles of "parentified child," "good child," and "symptomatic child" have been identified as having an impact in families in which there is adolescent drug abuse (Cleveland, 1981). Auxiliary roles of child "advocate," "analyst," "peacemaker," and "therapist" have also been described.

It is important for nurses to conceptualize the functional assessment category of roles in a family-oriented manner rather than an individual-oriented way.

> . . . the individual-oriented approach badly misrepresents the subject. For instance, to speak of the "role of the scapegoat" is to present the deviant as a person with fixed characteristics rather than a person involved in a process. "Scapegoating" technically applies to only one stage of a shifting scenario—the stage where the person is metaphorically cast out of the village. After all, the term originates from an ancient Hebrew ritual in which a goat was turned loose in the desert after the sins of the people had been symbolically laid on its head. The deviant can begin like a hero and go out like a villain, or vice versa. There is a positive-negative continuum on which he can be rated depending on which stage of the deviation process we are looking at, which sequence the process follows, and the degree to which the social system is stressed.
>
> At the time, the character of the deviant may vary in another direction, depending on the way his particular group does its typecasting. Which symptoms crop up in members of a group is itself a kind of typecasting. Thus the deviant may appear in many guises: the mascot, the clown, the sad sack, the erratic genius, the black sheep, the wise

guy, the saint, the idiot, the fool, the imposter, the malingerer, the boaster, the villain, and so on. Literature and folklore abound with such figures. (Hoffman, 1981, p. 58)

Questions to Ask the Family. To whom do most of you go when you need someone to talk to? What effect does it have on Brittany when Lamar helps with the baby's care? When Brittany and Lamar collaborate instead of competing, who would be the first to notice? If Lamar were to be more responsible for initiating contact with the relatives around the baby's day-care arrangements, how do you think Brittany would feel?

Influence

This subcategory refers to methods of affecting another's behavior. Instrumental influence or control refers to the use of objects or privileges as reinforcers (e.g., money, watching television, using the computer or telephone, candy, a vacation, and so forth). Psychological influence refers to the use of communication and feelings to influence behavior. Examples include directives, praise, criticism, and guilt induction. Corporal control refers to actual body contact such as hugging, spanking, and so forth. It is important to note the positive and negative influences used in the family, especially with infants and seniors. Abuse of seniors by informal caregivers is not infrequent.

Lytton (1980) found that the "most important positive predictors of compliance (for 2-year-old boys) are mother's consistency of enforcement of rules, her encouragement of mature action, her use of psychological rewards (praise and approval), and her play with the child. The most important negative one is the amount of physical punishment by mother" (p. 182). This finding is not surprising, for in our own clinical work we have found that the use of praise is positively related to compliance, whereas physical punishment and verbal, psychological punishment are constraining influences.

Questions to Ask the Family. Which of your parents is best at getting your sister to take her medication? When Armando dominates the conversation, what effect does that have on Anais? What does your mother feel about how your stepfather disciplines your sister? If your stepfather were to be more positive with your sister, how might his relationship with your mother change?

Beliefs

This subcategory refers to fundamental ideas, opinions, and assumptions held by individuals and families. Our beliefs are the blueprint from which we construct our lives. Families coevolve an ecology of beliefs that arise from interactional, social, and cultural contexts (Wright, et al. 1990). The nature of our beliefs can either increase or decrease our solution options when problems emerge (Watson & Lee, 1993; Wright & Nagy, 1993; Wright & Simpson, 1991; Wright & Watson, 1988; Wright, et al. 1990).

TABLE 3–5 BELIEFS ABOUT THE HEALTH PROBLEM

A. Beliefs about:
   1. Etiology
   2. Treatment
   3. Prognosis
   4. Role of healthcare professionals
   5. Role of the family
   6. Level of control the family has over the health problem

B. Influence of the family on the health problem
   1. Resource utilization
      a. Internal (to family)
      b. External
   2. Medication and treatment

C. Influence of the health problem on the family
   1. Client response to the illness
   2. Family members' responses to illness
   3. Perceived difficulties/changes related to the health problem

D. Strengths related to the health problem at present

E. Concerns related to the health problem at present

Adapted from Family Nursing Unit records, Faculty of Nursing, University of Calgary, Calgary, Alberta.

Cousins (1979) offered the poignant idea that what we believe is the most powerful option of all.

Beliefs and behavior are intricately connected. Every action, every choice families and individuals make, evolves from their beliefs. Consequently, beliefs shape the way families adapt to chronic and life-threatening illness. For example, if a family believes that the best treatment for colon cancer is a nontraditional approach, then it makes good sense if the family pursues acupuncture. Because our North American culture tends to use a paradigm of control about symptoms, it is very useful to explore family members' beliefs about control and mastery over their symptoms.

Table 3–5 provides a list of areas for nurses to explore when assessing family beliefs about the health problem.

Questions to Ask the Family. How much control do you believe your family has over chronic pain? How much control does chronic pain have over your family? What do you believe the effect would be, if any, on chronic pain if you and your wife agreed on treatment? What do you believe about you as a family that has enabled you to adapt so successfully to your chronic illness?

Alliances/Coalitions

This subcategory focuses on the directionality, balance, and intensity of relationships between family members or between families and nurses. Although _complementary_ and _symmetrical_ are terms employed to describe a two-person relationship (see Chapter 2), another term has been used to distinguish a three-person relationship. This term is *triangle*. The term was first coined by Murray Bowen (1978), a psychiatrist and family therapist, who explains:

> The two person relationship is unstable in that it has a low tolerance for anxiety and it is easily disturbed by emotional forces within the twosome and by relationship forces from outside the twosome. When anxiety increases, the emotional flow in a twosome intensifies and the relationship becomes uncomfortable. When the intensity reaches a certain level the twosome predictably and automatically involves a vulnerable third person in the emotional issue. The twosome might "reach out" and pull in the other person, the emotions might "over-flow" to the third person, or the third person might be emotionally programmed to initiate the involvement. With involvement of the third person, the anxiety level decreases. It is as if the anxiety is diluted as it shifts from one to another of the three relationships in a triangle. The triangle is more stable and flexible than the twosome. It has a much higher tolerance of anxiety and is capable of handling a fair percentage of life stresses. (p. 400)

Most family relationships are organized around threesomes or trian-gles. Relationships are not unidirectional even if one member of the triangle is an infant or an older person or has a handicap. The intensity of each relationship and the total amount of interaction is often fairly balanced. If one relationship becomes more intense, then another one or two become less intense. Also, if one member of a threesome withdraws, the other two become closer. We believe it is important for the nurse to note the degree of flexibility and fluidity within the family as they adjust to new arrivals, death, or illness.

As nurses assess this functional subcategory of alliances/coalitions, they will be aware of its interconnection with structural and developmen-tal categories. The structural subcategory of boundary is an important part of the alliance/coalition subcategory. The boundary defines who is part of the triangle and who is not. Of course, there are many triangles within families and many shifting alliances and coalitions. What is important to note, therefore, is the permeability of the boundary and whether the boundary crosses generations.

We have observed that crossgenerational coalitions sometimes coin-cide with symptomatic behavior. Hoffman (1981) has given an excellent example of a pattern of shifting crossgenerational triadic processes. The pattern focuses around the inappropriate behavior of a youngster:

> Stage one: Mother coaxes, child refuses to obey, mother threatens to tell father (father-mother against child). Stage two: when father comes home, mother tells him how bad child has been, and father sends child to his room without supper. Mother sneaks up after father has left the table and brings child a little food on a plate (mother-child against father). Stage three: when child comes down later, father, trying to

make up, offers to play a game with him that mother has expressly forbidden because it gets him too excited before bedtime (father-child against mother). Stage four: mother scolds father for this; the child, overexcited indeed, has a tantrum and is sent to bed; and the original triangle comes round again (mother-father against child). (p. 32)

In addition to noting the connection between the structural subcategory of boundary and the functional subcategory of alliances/coalitions, nurses should be aware of the interconnection with the developmental subcategory of attachments. A family's attachments, or underlying emotional bonds that have an enduring or stable quality, are similar to alliances in that they are both unions. Attachments tend to differ from coalitions, however, in that the latter imply an alignment between two members with a third member being split off or opposed.

Questions to Ask the Family. When Donald and Barbara argue, who is most likely to get in the middle of the fight? If the children are playing very well together, who would mostly likely come along and *start* them fighting? Who would *stop* them from fighting?

CONCLUSIONS

The CFAM is a "map of the family" from the nurse's observer perspective. The model provides a framework that can be drawn on as the nurse interviews the family. The nurse can use the three main categories (structural, developmental, and functional) to obtain a macro assessment of family strengths and problems. Depending on the nurse's confidence and competence level, she may do a more micro assessment and explore in detail specific areas of family functioning. In either situation, the nurse needs to be able to draw together all relevant information into an integrated assessment. It is insufficient to focus on a family's difficulties with problem-solving when the specific family structure is not known. Also, if the nurse focuses too much on previous developmental history, the nurse may be ignoring important current functioning issues. Naturally, past history cannot be ignored. It should be integrated, however, only insofar as it helps to explain current functioning.

Once a thorough family assessment has been completed, the nurse may now determine whether intervention is needed or not. However, we wish to emphasize that the completion of a family assessment utilizing CFAM does not mean that the nurse now has the "truth" about any particular family. Rather, the nurse has her own integrated assessment from her "observer perspective."

REFERENCES

Ahrons, C., & Rodgers, R. H. (1987). *Divorced families: A multidisciplinary developmental view.* New York: W. W. Norton.

Ashby, W. (1969). *Design for a brain.* London: Chapman & Hall, Science & Behavior Books.

Aylmer, R. (1988). The launching of the single young adult. In B. Carter & M.

McGoldrick (Eds.), *The changing family life cycle* (pp. 191–208). New York: Gardner Press.

Berenson, D. (1990). A systemic view of spirituality. *Journal of Strategic and Systemic Therapies, 9*(1), 59–70.

Bishop, D., Epstein, N., Baldwin, L., Miller, I., & Keitner, G. (1988). Older couples: The effect of health, retirement, and family functioning on morale. *Family Systems Medicine, 6*(2), 238–247.

Boss, P. (1980). Normative family stress: Family boundary changes across the life-span. *Family Relationships, 29*, 445–450.

Bowen, M. (1978). *Family therapy in clinical practice.* Northvale, NJ: Jason Aronson.

Bowlby, J. (1977). The making and breaking of affectional bonds. *British Journal of Psychiatry, 130*, 201–210.

Brown, F. H. (1988). The impact of death and serious illness on the family life cycle. In B. Carter & M. McGoldrick (Eds.), *The changing family life cycle: A framework for family therapy* (2nd ed., pp. 457–482). New York: Gardner Press.

Burns, L. H. (1987). Infertility as boundary ambiguity: One theoretical perspective. *Family Process, 26*(3), 359–372.

Carter, B., & McGoldrick, M. (Eds.). (1988). *The changing family life cycle: A framework for family therapy* (2nd ed.). New York: Gardner Press.

Cheng-Ham, M. D. (1989). Family therapy with immigrant families: Constructing a bridge between different world views. *Journal of Strategic and Systemic Therapies, 8*,1–2.

Cleveland, M. (1981). Families and adolescent drug abuse: Structural analysis of children's roles. *Family Process, 20*,295–304.

Cousins, N. (1979). *Anatomy of an illness as perceived by the patient.* New York: Bantam Books.

Duvall, E. (1977). *Marriage and family development* (5th ed.). Philadelphia: J. B. Lippincott.

Divorce rate drops. (1991, August). *Family Therapy News*, p. 16.

Epstein, N., Bishop, D., & Levin, S. (1978). The McMaster model of family functioning. *Journal of Marriage and Family Counseling, 4*, 19–31.

Epstein, N., Sigal, J., & Rakoff, V. (1968). *Family categories schema.* Unpublished manuscript, Jewish General Hospital, Department of Psychiatry, Montreal.

Ericksen, J., Yancey, W., & Ericksen, E. (1979). The division of family roles. *Journal of Marriage and the Family, 41*, 301–313.

Erickson, E. (1963). *Childhood and society* (2nd ed.). New York: W. W. Norton.

Falicov, C. J. (1988). Family sociology and family therapy contributions to the family development framework: A comparative analysis and thoughts on future trends. In C. J. Falivoc (Ed.), *Family transitions: Continuity and change over the life cycle* (pp. 3–54). New York: Guilford Press.

Fulmer, R. (1988). Lower-income and professional families: A comparison of structure and life cycle process. In B. Carter & M. McGoldrick (Eds.), *The changing family life cycle* (pp. 545–578). New York: Gardner Press.

Giordano, J. (1988). Parents of the baby boomers: A new generation of young-old. *Family Relations, 37*, 411–414.

Glick, P. C. (1989a). The family life cycle and social change. *Family Relations, 38*, 123–129.

Glick, P. (1989b). Remarried families, stepfamilies, and stepchildren: A brief demographic profile. *Family Relations, 38*, 24–27.

Goldner, V. (1988). Generation and gender: Normative and covert hierarchies. *Family Process, 27*, 17–32.

Gross, J. (1992, March 29). Collapse of inner-city families creates America's new orphans. *The New York Times*, pp. 1, 15.

Hagestad, G. O. (1988). Demographic change and the life course: Some emerging trends in the family realm. *Family Relations, 37,* 405–410.

Hajal, F., & Rosenberg, E. (1991). The family life cycle in adoptive families. *American Journal of Orthopsychiatry, 61*(1), 78–85.

Haley, J. (1977). Toward a theory of pathological systems. In P. Watzlawick & J. Weakland (Eds.), *The interactional view.* New York: W. W. Norton.

Hampson, R. B., Beavers, W. R., & Hulgus, Y. (1990). Cross-ethnic family differences: Interactional assessment of white, black and Mexican-American families. *Journal of Marital and Family Therapy, 16*(3), 307–319.

Hanson, S. M. H., & Bozett, F. (1986). The changing nature of fatherhood: The nurse and social policy. *Journal of Advanced Nursing, 11,* 719–727.

Hardy, K. V. (1990, September/October). Much more than techniques needed in treating minorities. *Family Therapy News*

Hartman, A. (1978). Diagrammatic assessment of family relationships. *Social Casework, 59,* 465–476.

Healy, J., Malley, J., & Stewart, A. (1990). Children and their fathers after parental separation. *American Journal of Orthopsychiatry, 60*(4), 531–543.

Hill, R. (1986). Life cycle stages for types of single-parent families: Of family development theory. *Family Relations, 35,* 19–29.

Hines, P. M. (1988). The family life cycle of poor black families. In B. Carter & M. McGoldrick (Eds.), *The changing family life cycle* (pp. 513–544). New York: Gardner Press.

Hoffman, L. (1981). *Foundations of family therapy.* New York: Basic Books.

Imber-Black, E. (1991). The family-larger system perspective. *Family Systems Medicine, 9*(4), 371–396.

Leahey, M., & Wright, L. M. (Eds.). (1987a). *Families and life-threatening illness.* Springhouse, PA: Springhouse.

Leahey, M., & Wright, L. M. (Eds.). (1987b). *Families and psychosocial problems.* Springhouse, PA: Springhouse.

Lewis, J. (1988a). The transition to parenthood: 1. The rating of prenatal marital competence. *Family Process, 27*(2), 149–166.

Lewis, J. (1988b). The transition to parenthood: 2. Stability and change in marital structure. *Family Process, 27*(3), 273–284.

Lewis, J., Owen, M. T., & Cox, M. (1988). The transition to parenthood: 3. Incorporation of the child into the family. *Family Process 27*(4), 411–421.

Lupri, E., & Frideres, J. (1981). The quality of marriage and the passage of time: Marital satisfaction over the family life cycle. *Canadian Journal of Sociology, 6,* 283–305.

Lytton, H. (1980). *Parent-child interaction: The socialization process observed in twin and singleton families.* New York: Plenum Press.

McGoldrick, M. (1982). Normal families: An ethnic perspective. In F. Walsh (Ed.), *Normal family processes* (pp. 399–424). New York: Guilford Press.

McGoldrick, M. (1988a). Ethnicity and the family life cycle. In B. Carter & M. McGoldrick (Eds.), *The changing family life cycle* (pp. 69–90). New York: Gardner Press.

McGoldrick, M. (1988b). Women and the family life cycle. In B. Carter & M. McGoldrick (Eds.), *The changing family life cycle* (pp. 29–68). New York: Gardner Press.

McGoldrick, M. (1991). Echoes from the past: Helping families mourn their losses. In F. Walsh & M. McGoldrick (Eds.), *Living beyond loss: Death in the family* (pp. 50–78). New York: W. W. Norton.

McGoldrick, M., & Gerson, R. (1985). *Genograms in family assessment.* New York: W. W. Norton.

McGoldrick, M., & Gerson, R. (1988). Genograms and the family life cycle. In B.

Carter & M. McGoldrick (Eds.), *The changing family life cycle* (pp. 164–189). New York: Gardner Press.

Minuchin, S. (1974). *Families and family therapy.* Cambridge, MA: Harvard University Press.

Pallett, P. (1990). A conceptual framework for studying family caregiver burden in Alzheimer's type dementia. *Image, 22*(1), 52–58.

Parenthood II: The nest won't stay empty. (1989, March 12). *The New York Times,* pp. 1, 22.

Parks, S. H., & Pilisuk, M. (1991). Caregiver burden: Gender and the psychological costs of caregiving. *American Journal of Orthopsychiatry, 61*(4), 501–509.

Parsons, T., & Bales, R. (1956). *Family: Socialization and interaction process.* London: Routledge & Kegan Paul.

Pill, C. (1990). Stepfamilies: Redefining the family. *Family Relations, 39,* 186–193.

Quinn, P., & Allen, K. (1989). Facing challenges and making compromises: How single mothers endure. *Family Relations, 38,* 390–395.

Reitz, M., & Watson, K. W. (1992). *Adoption and the family system.* New York: Guilford Press.

Schibuk, M. (1989). Treating the sibling subsystem: An adjunct of divorce therapy. *American Journal of Orthopsychiatry, 59*(2), 226–237.

Schnittger, M., & Bird, G. (1990). Coping among dual-career men and women across the family life cycle. *Family Relations, 39,* 199–205.

Selvini, M., Boscolo, L., Cecchin, G., & Prata, G. (1989). Hypothesizing—circularity—neutrality: Three guidelines for the conduction of the session. *Family Process, 19*(1), 3–12.

Sheinberg, M., & Penn, P. (1991). Gender dilemmas, gender questions, and the gender mantra. *Journal of Marital and Family Therapy, 17*(1), 33–44.

Simon, R. (1988). Family life cycle issues in the therapy system. In B. Carter & M. McGoldrick (Eds.), *The changing family life cycle: A framework for family therapy* (2nd ed., pp. 107–118). New York: Gardner Press.

Stuart, M. (1991). An analysis of the concept of family. In A. Whall & J. Fawcett (Eds.), *Family theory development in nursing: State of the science and art* (pp. 31–42). Philadelphia: F. A. Davis.

Suro, R. (1991, December 29). The new American family: Reality is wearing the pants. *The New York Times,* Section 4, p. 2.

Terkelson, K. (1980). Toward a theory of the family life cycle. In B. Carter & M. McGoldrick (Eds.), *The family life cycle: A framework for family therapy* (pp. 21–52). New York: Gardner Press.

Toman, W. (1976). *Family constellation: Its effects on personality and social behavior* (3rd ed.). New York: Springer.

Toman, W. (1988). Basics of family structure and sibling position. In M. D. Kahn & K. G. Lewis (Eds.), *Siblings in therapy: Life span and clinical issues* (pp. 46–65). New York: W. W. Norton.

Tomm, K. (1977). *Tripartite family assessment.* Unpublished manuscript, University of Calgary, Alberta.

Tomm, K. (1980). Towards a cybernetic systems approach to family therapy at the University of Calgary. In D. Freeman (Ed.), *Perspectives on family therapy* (pp. 3–18). Vancouver: Butterworth.

Tomm, K., & Sanders, G. (1983). Family assessment in a problem oriented record. In J. C. Hansen & B. F. Keeney (Eds.), *Diagnosis and assessment in family therapy* (pp. 101–122). London: Aspen Systems.

Waldegrave, C. (1990). Just therapy. *Dulwich Centre Newsletter, 1,* 5–46.

Walsh, F., & McGoldrick, M. (Eds.). (1991). *Living beyond loss: Death in the family.* New York: W. W. Norton.

Watson, W. L., & Lee, D. (1993). Is there life after suicide? The systemic belief approach for "survivors" of suicide. *Archives of Psychiatric Nursing, 6*(1).

Watzlawick, P., Beavin, J., & Jackson, D. (1967). *Pragmatics of human communication.* New York: W. W. Norton.

Westley, W., & Epstein, N. (1969). *The silent majority.* San Francisco: Jossey-Bass.

White, M. (1991). Deconstruction and therapy. *Dulwich Centre Newsletter, 3,* 21–40.

Wright, L. M., & Leahey, M. (Eds.). (1987). *Families and chronic illness.* Springhouse, PA: Springhouse.

Wright, L. M., & Nagy, J. (1993). Death: The most troublesome family secret of all. In E. Imber-Black (Ed.), *Secrets in families and family therapy* (pp. 121–137). New York: W. W. Norton.

Wright, L. M., & Simpson, P. (1991). A systemic belief approach to epileptic seizures: A case of being spellbound. *Contemporary Family Therapy: An International Journal, 13*(2), 165–180.

Wright, L. M., & Watson, W. L. (1988). Systemic family therapy and family development. In C. J. Falicov (Ed.), *Family transitions: Continuity and change over the life cycle* (pp. 407–430). New York: Guilford Press.

Wright, L. M., Watson, W. L., & Bell, J. M. (1990). The Family Nursing Unit: A unique integration of research, education and clinical practice. In J. M. Bell, W. L. Watson, & L. M. Wright (Eds.), *The cutting edge of family nursing* (pp. 95–109). Calgary, Alberta: Family Nursing Unit Publications.

THE CALGARY FAMILY INTERVENTION MODEL

The Calgary Family Intervention Model (CFIM) is a companion model to the Calgary Family Assessment Model (CFAM) (Chapter 3). Over the past 20 years, several family assessment models and family measurement instruments have been developed by both nurses and others (Mischke-Berkey, Warner, & Hanson, 1989). To our knowledge, CFIM is the first family intervention model to emerge within nursing. We make reference to this development to punctuate another milestone in nurses' efforts to put into language the important involvement they have with families.

This chapter presents our definition and description of CFIM, examples of interventions at three domains of family functioning, and actual clinical examples using CFIM. We conclude this chapter with intervention ideas for common family situations nurses encounter.

DEFINITION AND DESCRIPTION

After a comprehensive family assessment has been completed and family intervention is indicated, the nurse needs to consider where she desires to trigger a perturbation to encourage change. CFIM is an organizing framework for conceptualizing the intersection between a particular domain of family functioning and the specific intervention offered by the nurse (Table 4–1). CFIM visually portrays the "fit" between a domain of family functioning and a nursing intervention; that is, does the intervention effect change in the domain or not? The elements of CFIM are interventions, domains of family functioning, and "fit" or effectiveness. CFIM is focused on promoting, improving, and/or sustaining effective family functioning in three domains: cognitive, affective, and behavioral. We identified these three domains in our 1984 edition of this book but now have incorporated them into CFIM.

Interventions can be targeted to promote, improve, or sustain functioning at any or all of the three domains of family functioning, but a

TABLE 4–1 CALGARY FAMILY INTERVENTION MODEL (CFIM): INTERSECT OF
DOMAINS OF FAMILY FUNCTIONING AND INTERVENTIONS

		Interventions Offered by Nurse
Domains of Family Functioning	**Cognitive**	**"Fit" or Effectiveness**
	Affective	
	Behavioral	

change in one domain will have an impact on another domain. However, we believe that the most profound and sustaining change will be that which occurs within the family's beliefs (cognition). In other words, as a family thinketh, they are so. One intervention could actually target cognitive, affective, and behavioral domains of family functioning simultaneously. A significant determining factor is if the intervention is selected as a trigger (perturbation) for potential change by the family. We believe nurses can only *offer* interventions to the family. Whether the family opens space for an intervention depends on its genetic make up and its history of interactions between family members. This decision also is profoundly influenced by the relationship between the nurse and the family (Thorne & Robinson, 1989) and by the nurse's ability to invite the family to reflect on its health problems (Wright & Levac, 1992). Second-order cybernetics and the work of Maturana (Maturana & Varela, 1992) have influenced our ideas in this regard (Chapter 2).

Intervening in a family system in a manner that will promote or facilitate change is the most challenging and exciting aspect of clinical work with families. The intervention stage represents the core of clinical practice with families. It provides an appropriate context in which the family can make necessary changes. There are a myriad of interventions that the nurse could choose, but nurses need to tailor their interventions to each family and to the chosen domain of family functioning. Particular interventions will generally vary for each family, although there may be occasions when the same intervention is used for several families and for different problems. However, we wish to emphasize that each family is unique and that even though labeling particular interventions is of great importance for putting our practice into language, it does not represent a cookbook approach. The interventions we list are *examples* of interventions that could be used, and they are not intended to be all inclusive. We have given examples of interventions that we have found from our clinical practice and research to be very useful. The interventions that we cite are based on several important theoretical foundations: systems, cybernetics, communication, and change theory (Chapter 2).

In summary, CFIM is neither a list of nursing interventions nor a list of family functioning. Rather, it provides a means to conceptualize a fit between domains of family functioning and interventions offered by the nurse. It assists in determining the predominant domain of family functioning that needs changing and the most useful intervention that will effect change in that domain. Through therapeutic conversations, the family and nurse collaborate and coevolve to discover the most useful fit. We use the qualitative term "fit" in a slightly different way than de Shazer (1988) does, as we emphasize whether or not the interventions effect change in the presenting problem. Fit involves a recognition of reciprocity between the nurse's ideas and opinions and the family's illness experience. Therefore, determining fit may involve some experimentation or trial and error. It also entails a belief by nurses that each family is unique and has particular strengths. In Chapter 7 we outline factors to enhance the likelihood that interventions will trigger change in the desired domain of family functioning.

INTERVENTIVE QUESTIONS

One of the simplest but most powerful nursing interventions for families experiencing health problems is the use of interventive questions. Interventive questions are intended to actively effect change in any one or all three of the domains. Nurses conducting family interviews should remember, though, that knowledge of when, how, and to what purpose to pose questions is more important than simply choosing one type of question over another (Lipchik & de Shazer, 1986).

LINEAR VERSUS CIRCULAR QUESTIONS

Interventive questions are usually of two types: linear or circular. (Tomm, 1987, 1988). Linear questions tend to inform the nurse, whereas circular questions are meant to effect change (Tomm, 1985; Tomm, 1987, 1988). The important difference between these kinds of questions is their intent. Linear questions are investigative; they explore a family member's perceptions and descriptions of a problem. For example, when exploring family members' perceptions of their daughter's anorexia nervosa, the nurse would begin with linear questions: "When did you notice that your daughter had changed her eating habits?" "What do you think caused your daughter to stop eating as she normally would?" These linear questions, while informing the nurse of the history of the young woman's eating patterns, also help illuminate family perceptions or beliefs about eating patterns. Linear questions are frequently used to begin gathering information about families' problems, whereas circular questions reveal families' understanding of problems.

Circular questions are directed toward explanations of problems. For example, of the same family the nurse could ask, "Who in the family is most worried about Cheyenne's anorexia?" "How does Mother show that she's the one worrying the most?" Circular questions help the nurse to discover valuable information because these questions seek out relationships between individuals, events, ideas, and beliefs.

The effect of these questions on families is quite distinct. Linear questions tend to be constraining, whereas circular questions are generative; the latter introduce new cognitive connections, paving the way for new or different family behaviors. The linear form of questioning implies that the nurse knows what is best for the family; it also implies that she has become purposive and invested in a particular outcome. Linear questions are intended to correct behavior; circular questions are intended to facilitate behavioral change.

The primary distinction between circular and lineal questions lies in the notion that information reveals differences in relationships (Bateson, 1979). With circular questions, a relationship or connection is always sought between individuals, events, ideas, and beliefs. With linear questions, the focus is cause and effect. The idea of circular questions evolved from the concept of circularity and the method of circular interviewing developed by the originators of Milan Systemic Family Therapy (Fleuridas, Nelson, & Rosenthal, 1986; Selvini-Palazzoli, Boscolo, Cecchin, & Prata, 1980; Tomm, 1984, 1985, 1987) (Chapters 6 and 7). Circularity involves the cycle of questions and answers between families and nurses that occurs during the interview process. The nurse's questions are based on information that the family gives in response to the questions the nurse asks, and thus the cycle continues (Watson, 1992). The family's responses to the questions provide information for the nurse and the family. The questions in and of themselves also provide new information and answers for the family. This is when they are considered interventions. Interventive questions may invite family members to see their problems in a new way and subsequently to see new solutions. Thus, as the family's answers provide information for the nurse, the nurse's questions may provide information for the family (Watson, 1992).

Tomm (1987) embellished the types of circular questions utilized by the Milan Systemic Family Therapy team and identified, defined, and classified various circular questions. Loos and Bell (1990) creatively applied the use of circular questions to critical care nursing. Watson (1988a, 1988b, 1988c, 1989a, 1989b) demonstrated the therapeutic aspect of circular questions with families experiencing chronic illness, life-threatening illness, and psychosocial problems. The circular questions identified by Tomm (1987) that we have found most useful in clinical practice with families are difference questions, behavioral effect questions, hypothetical/future-oriented questions, and triadic questions. We have expanded the use of circular questions by providing examples of questions that can be asked to intervene in the cognitive, affective, and behavioral domains of family functioning. The various types of questions, definitions, and examples are given in Table 4–2.

TABLE 4–2 CIRCULAR QUESTIONS TO CHANGE COGNITIVE, AFFECTIVE, AND BEHAVIORAL DOMAINS OF FAMILY FUNCTIONING

1. Type: Difference Question
Definition: Explores differences between people, relationships, time, ideas, and beliefs.
Examples of intervening at three domains of family functioning:

Cognitive	*Affective*	*Behavioral*
• What's the best advice that you've had about managing your son's AIDS? What's the worst advice?	• Who in the family is most worried about how AIDS is transmitted?	• Who's the best in the family at getting your son to take his medication on time?
• What information would be most helpful to you about managing the effects of sexual abuse? Who in the family would benefit most with more information?	• Who is finding your disclosure of sexual abuse most difficult?	• When you first disclosed your sexual abuse, what was done by professionals that was most helpful?

2. Type: Behavioral Effect Question
Definition: Explores connections between the effect of one family member's behavior on another.
Examples of intervening at three domains of family functioning:

Cognitive	*Affect*	*Behavioral*
• How do you make sense of your husband not visiting your son in hospital?	• What do you feel when your son cries following his treatments?	• What do you do when your husband doesn't visit your son in the hospital?
• What do you know about the effect of life-threatening illness on children?	• How does your mother show she is afraid of dying?	• What could your father do that indicates to your mother that he understands her fears?

3. Type: Hypothetical/Future-Oriented Question
Definition: Explores family options and alternative actions or meanings in the future.
Examples of intervening at three domains of family functioning:

Cognitive	*Affective*	*Behavioral*
• What do you think will happen if these skin grafts continue to be so painful for your son?	• If your son's skin grafts aren't successful, what do you think his mood will be? Sad? Mad? Resigned?	• How much longer will it be before your son may invite himself to accept treatment for his contractures?
• If the worst scenario occurred, how do you think your family would cope?	• If things don't go well with your grandmother's treatment, who will be most affected?	• How long do you think your grandmother will have to remain in the hospital? If it's longer, what do you think your brothers and sisters will do?
• If you did decide to have your grandmother institutionalized, who would you discuss it with?		

Continued on following page

4. Type: Triadic Question

Definition: Question posed to a third person about the relationship between two other people.

Examples of intervening at three domains of family functioning:

Cognitive	Affective	Behavioral
• If your father were not drinking daily, what would your mother think about him going to the rehab center?	• What does your father do that invites your mother to be less anxious about his condition?	• If your father were willing to talk with your mother about solutions to his addiction problem, what could he say?
• How does your dad know that your sister needs support?	• When your dad supports your sister, how does your mom feel?	• What do you think your father needs to do to prepare for your sister's long treatment?

In summary, the four types of circular questions (difference, behavioral effect, hypothetical, and triadic) can be used to trigger change in any one or all of the domains of family functioning. Table 4–3 illustrates the intersect of various types of circular questions and the domains of family functioning. We wish to emphasize strongly that what is most critical is the effectiveness/usefulness/fit of the question in triggering change, rather than the specific question itself.

OTHER EXAMPLES OF INTERVENTIONS

To illustrate the intersection of three domains of family functioning (cognitive, affective, and behavioral) and various interventions we have chosen several other examples of interventions in addition to circular questions. These examples are not meant to be an exhaustive list. Rather, they are interventions we have found useful in our own clinical practice and research.

TABLE 4–3 INTERSECTION OF CIRCULAR QUESTIONS AND DOMAINS OF FAMILY FUNCTIONING

		Interventions Offered by Nurse: Circular Questions			
		Difference	**Behavioral Effect**	**Hypothetical**	**Triadic**
Domains of Family Functioning	Cognitive				
	Affective				
	Behavioral				

TABLE 4–4 INTERSECTION OF INTERVENTION (OFFERING INFORMATION)
AND DOMAINS OF FAMILY FUNCTIONING

		Intervention: Offering Information
Domains of Family Functioning	Cognitive	
	Affective	
	Behavioral	

The examples include:

- Commending family and individual strengths
- Offering information/opinions
- Reframing
- Offering education
- Externalizing the problem
- Validating/normalizing emotional responses
- Storying the illness experience
- Drawing forth family support
- Encouraging family members as caregivers
- Encouraging respite
- Devising rituals

These interventions can trigger change in any one or all of the domains of family functioning. For example, the nurse can use the intervention of offering information to promote change in cognitive, affective, or behavioral family functioning (Table 4–4).

A description of each intervention and a case example illustrating its application follows.

We have chosen to cluster the sample interventions around a particular domain of family functioning. In doing this, we do not wish to imply that one intervention can only be used to trigger change in one domain of family functioning. We also do not want to imply that one intervention is a "cognitive intervention" and another an "affective intervention." Rather, these are examples of the fit between a specific problem, a particular intervention, and a domain of family functioning.

INTERVENTIONS TO CHANGE THE COGNITIVE DOMAIN OF FAMILY FUNCTIONING

Interventions directed at the cognitive domain of family functioning are usually those that give new ideas, opinions, information, or education on a particular health problem or risk. The treatment goal or desired outcome is to change how a particular family perceives and believes with regard to its health problem so that members can discover new solutions to their health problems. We offer the following interventions as examples to change the cognitive domain of family functioning.

COMMENDING FAMILY AND INDIVIDUAL STRENGTHS

We routinely commend families in each session on the strengths observed during the interview. Commendations differ from compliments. de Shazer (1988) describes compliments as statements from the interviewer "about what the client has said that is useful, effective, good, or fun" with the purpose of promoting cooperation on the task at hand (p. 96). Commendations are observations of patterns of behavior that occur across time (e.g., "Your family members are very loyal to one another") whereas a compliment is usually an observational comment on a one-time event (e.g., "you were very praising of your son today"). Families coping with chronic, life-threatening, or psychosocial problems frequently feel defeated, hopeless, and like failures in their efforts to overcome their illnesses or to live with them satisfactorily. Commonly, families coping with health problems have not been commended for their strengths or even made aware of them (McElheran & Harper-Jaques, 1994). The immediate and long-term positive reactions to such commendations indicate that they are effective therapeutic actions. Families who internalize commendations appear more receptive to other therapeutic actions that may be offered.

In one family, an adopted son's behavioral and emotional problems had kept members involved with healthcare professionals for 10 years. The nurse commended this family by telling members that she believed they were the best family for this boy because many other families would not have been as sensitive to his needs and would probably have given up years ago. Both parents became tearful and said that this was the first positive statement made to them as parents in many years.

By commending families' competence and strengths, and offering them a new opinion of themselves, a context for change is created that allows families to then discover their own solutions to problems. By changing the view they have of themselves, families are frequently able to view the health problem differently and thus move toward more effective solutions.

OFFERING INFORMATION/OPINIONS

Families with a hospitalized member have indicated that a high priority is the obtaining of information. Many families have expressed to us their frustration at their inability to obtain information or opinions readily from healthcare professionals. Nurses can offer to provide information about the impact of chronic or life-shortening illnesses on families. Nurses also can empower *families* to obtain information about resources. We have learned that this latter approach is even more useful in some circumstances.

One clinical example concerns a family of two aging parents and their 34-year-old son with severe multiple sclerosis. The parents were constant, devoted caretakers but had not had any respite for several months. The son was asked by the nurse if he would be willing to challenge his belief about himself as being "helpless." The nurse asked him to take the leadership role in exploring possible resources for caregivers so that his parents might have a vacation. As a result of his search, the son discovered he was eligible for many financial benefits of which he had previously been unaware, including benefits to hire professional caregivers. Shortly afterward, the son made arrangements for 24-hour in-home nursing care while his parents took a vacation. His parents reported that they felt much less stressed and their son was also much happier. He began making efforts to walk using parallel bars, an activity that he had not done in several months.

In this case example, the nurse offered an opinion to empower the son to change his cognitive set. The intervention fit the cognitive domain, and results also took place in the affective and behavioral domains of family functioning.

REFRAMING

According to Watzlawick, Weakland, and Fisch (1974), reframing changes the conceptual and/or emotional setting or viewpoint in relation to which a situation is experienced and places it in another frame, which fits the "facts" of the same concrete situation equally well or even better and thereby changes its meaning.

The problem is thus lifted out of the symptom frame and placed in a frame that implies change. The symptom is given another meaning. Jessee and colleagues (1982) describe the use of positive reframing with hospitalized school children and suggest that reframing has implications for the child's interpersonal development. "Perhaps most significant is that reframing may affect both the emotional and conceptual aspects of the child's self-evaluation" (Jessee, Jurkovic, Wilkie, & Chiglinski, 1982, p. 314). They experienced significant success with the use of reframing interventions to effect behavioral change.

OFFERING EDUCATION

Helping parents to understand and help their children (Craft & Willadsen, 1992) is a common but important intervention for families. Nurses can teach about normal physiological, emotional, and cognitive characteristics as well as identify developmental tasks or goals of children and adolescents that can be affected or altered during times of illness (Craft & Willadsen, 1992; Duhamel, 1987). One family found it very useful to have the nurse explain that siblings of children experiencing life-shortening illnesses often develop symptoms due to feelings of loneliness because parents are intently focused on their ill child.

EXTERNALIZING THE PROBLEM

A very innovative intervention, which was developed by Michael White of Australia, is the externalization of a problem (Tomm, 1989; White, 1984, 1986, 1988–1989; White & Epston, 1989). This involves separating the problem from the personal identity of the client. Instead of viewing the problem as residing in the person, the problem is externalized and viewed as being outside the person. Rather than a client's being objectified, a problem is objectified (White, 1988–1989). Externalization can be achieved during a family interview by introducing questions that encourage family members to map the influence of the problem in their lives and their influence in the life of the problem. This is called relative influence questioning (White, 1988). The family is asked, "How much influence do you have over the problem?" and reciprocally, "How much influence does the problem have over you and your relationship?" The following dialogue between the nurse and a husband whose young wife was experiencing epileptic seizures illustrates how a new description of the problem is coevolved by externalizing the seizures (Wright & Simpson, 1991).

Nurse: The spells [the young woman referred to the seizures as spells] are so intrusive and rude, they seem to take control of the whole situation.

Husband: Oh, yeah, it happens all the time.

Nurse: Is there anything you've done that helps to gain more control of them?

Husband: I've tried everything.

Nurse: It seems that everyone is at their mercy.

Husband: Yes, they happen anywhere, anytime.

Relative influence questioning (White, 1988) elucidated the influence this couple had over the impact of seizures on their lives and contrasted it with the amount of influence the seizures had in controlling the couple. This created a double description (White, 1986). The couple could now view the problem from two perspectives rather than one.

We have also externalized chronic pain, phobias, and depressions, with dramatic, positive results with adults. Externalization of the problem is also particularly useful with children experiencing phobias, encopresis, enuresis, behavioral problems, and chronic pain. Externalizing the problem was even useful with a teenager who was experiencing depression related to her jealous feelings about a friend who reminded her of Marilyn Monroe. In this case, the problem was externalized as "a case of Marilynitis" and had a very positive outcome (Wright & Park Dorsay, 1989).

INTERVENTIONS TO CHANGE THE AFFECTIVE DOMAIN OF FAMILY FUNCTIONING

Interventions aimed at the affective domain of family functioning are designed to reduce or increase intense emotions that may be blocking families' problem-solving efforts. Following are examples of interventions that can change the affective domain of family functioning.

VALIDATING/NORMALIZING EMOTIONAL RESPONSES

Validation of intense affect can alleviate feelings of isolation and loneliness and assist family members to make the connection between a family member's illness and their emotional responses. For example, following a diagnosis of a life-shortening illness, families frequently feel out of control or frightened for a period of time. It is important for nurses to validate these strong emotions and to reassure and offer hope to families that in time they will adjust and learn ways to cope.

STORYING THE ILLNESS EXPERIENCE

Too often family members are only encouraged to tell the medical story or narrative of their illness rather than the story of their *experience* of their illness. Through therapeutic conversations, nurses can create a trusting environment for the open expression of family members' fears, anger, and sadness about their illness experience. Having an opportunity to express the impact of the illness on the family and the influence of the family on the illness from each family member's perspective gives validation to the experience. This is very different from limiting or constraining family stories to symptoms, medication, and physical treatments. By having a context provided for the sharing of the illness experience between family members, intense emotions are legitimized.

DRAWING FORTH FAMILY SUPPORT

Nurses can enhance family functioning in the affective domain through providing and assisting family members to listen to each other's concerns and feelings (Craft & Willadsen, 1992). This can be particularly useful at times when a family member may be dying or has died. Through fostering opportunities for family members to express this painful experience, the nurse can enable the family members to draw forth their own strengths and resources to support one another. Nurses can be the catalyst to facilitate communication between family members or between the family and other healthcare professionals. This type of family support can prevent families from becoming unduly burdened or defeated by an illness.

INTERVENTIONS TO CHANGE THE BEHAVIORAL DOMAIN OF FAMILY FUNCTIONING

Interventions directed at the behavioral domain assist family members to behave differently in relation to one another. This change is most often accomplished by inviting some or all family members to engage in specific behavioral tasks. Some tasks are given during a family meeting so that the nurse can observe the interaction, while others may be experimented with between sessions. Sometimes, it is necessary for the nurse to review with the family what the particular task and experiment is in order to check the family's understanding of what has been suggested.

We offer the following examples of interventions that could change the behavioral domain of family functioning.

ENCOURAGING FAMILY MEMBERS TO BE CAREGIVERS

Family members are often timid or afraid to become involved in the care of their ill family member unless supported by a nurse to do so. Our experience has been that family members very much appreciate an opportunity to be *doing* something for their hospitalized family member as a way of feeling a sense of helpfulness and control.

ENCOURAGING RESPITE

Often, it is very difficult for caretaking family members to allow themselves adequate respite. Too frequently, family members feel guilty if they need or want to withdraw themselves from the caregiving role. Even the ill member must disengage him or herself from time to time from the usual caregiver and accept another person's assistance. Each family's need for respite varies. The issues affecting respite requirements include the severity of the chronic illness and the availability of financial resources and family members to care for the ill person (Leahey & Wright, 1987). All of these issues must be considered before a nurse recommends a respite schedule. Tucker (1984) reports that she advises families to buy a less expensive prosthesis and use the extra money for a family vacation. In this way, caregiving and coping are balanced. Such "time outs" or "time away" are essential for families facing excessive caretaking demands. Another example is to recommend to a mother and father with a leukemic child to have grandparents babysit for a day while the couple have time together.

DEVISING RITUALS

Families engage in many daily rituals (e.g., bedtime reading), yearly rituals (e.g., Thanksgiving dinner at Grandma's), and cultural rituals (e.g., ethnic parades). Nurses can suggest therapeutic rituals that are not or have not been observed by the family. Roberts (1988) defines rituals as

> coevolved symbolic acts that include not only the ceremonial aspects of the actual presentation of the ritual, but the process of preparing for

it as well. It may or may not include words, but does have both open and closed parts which are "held" together by a guiding metaphor. Repetition can be a part of rituals through either the content, the form, or the occasion. There should be enough space in therapeutic rituals for the incorporation of multiple meanings by various family members and clinicians, as well as a variety of levels of participation. (p. 8)

In our clinical practice, we have observed that chronic illness and psychosocial problems frequently interrupt usual rituals. Rituals are best introduced when there is an excessive level of confusion caused by the simultaneous presentation of incompatible injunctions. Rituals serve to provide clarity in a family system (Imber-Black, Roberts, & Whiting, 1988). For example, parents who cannot agree on parenting practices often end up giving conflicting messages to their families. This can result in chaos and confusion for their children. The introduction of an odd-day, even-day ritual (Selvini-Palazzoli, et al. 1978) can often assist the family. The mother could be invited to experiment with being responsible for the children on Mondays, Wednesdays, and Fridays, and the father on Tuesdays, Thursdays, and Saturdays. On Sundays, they could behave spontaneously. On their "days off," parents could be asked to observe, without comment, their partner's parenting. This intervention isolates contradictory behaviors by prescribing sequence (Tomm, 1984).

CLINICAL CASE EXAMPLES

Actual clinical case examples follow to illustrate the utilization of CFIM. Interventions were chosen to trigger change in all three domains of family functioning.

CLINICAL CASE EXAMPLE 1

To illustrate a particular family intervention aimed at all three domains of family functioning (cognitive, affective, and behavioral) simultaneously, let us consider a common parenting problem presented to community health nurses (CHNs). The problem is of young parents who are having difficulty putting their 3-year-old son to bed each night. Their efforts are always met with a hassle from their son, then anger, then tears. In their efforts, the parents also become very frustrated and frequently end up angry with each other as well as with their son.

It is to be emphasized that it is not always necessary or even efficient to try to fit target interventions to all *three* domains of family functioning simultaneously. Again, this will depend on how well the family is engaged and the assessment of the nature of the problems.

With this particular problem of parents' chronic inability to have their 3-year-old son go to bed at a required time and stay in bed, the family intervention offered was parent education. This intervention is defined as helping parents to understand and help their young children (Craft &

Willadsen, 1992). In describing this case example, we also discuss particular executive skills the nurse can use to operationalize the intervention.

Parent-Child System Problem: Parents' chronic inability to have 3-year-old son go to bed at a required time and stay in bed.

Domains of Family Functioning	*Intervention: Parent education*
Cognitive	Offer a parenting book for ideas on what bedtime means to children and how to put children to bed.
Affective	Inform the parents that it is important to admit their frustrations to one another, especially if one spouse made an effort to put the child to bed but has not been successful. The other parent may give emotional support (e.g., "You tried real hard, dear; he's a handful").
Behavioral	Teach the parents that when they put their son to bed, they should not respond to his efforts to gain attention (e.g., asking for a glass of water). Rather, be sure that these things have been attended to as part of his bedtime ritual. Prepare parents that to extinguish their child's behavior of continually calling them to his bedroom or coming out of his room, they must accept that his behavior will worsen for a few nights while he makes greater efforts to get his parents to respond. Then, if the parents continue in a very matter-of-fact way to put him back in his room and tell him "no" to any further requests, his behavior will probably dramatically improve in a few nights.

CLINICAL CASE EXAMPLE 2

Next, let us consider a clinical example illustrating the utilization of the interventions of encouraging family members to be caregivers and caregiver support. Encouraging family members to be caregivers is the inviting of family members to be involved in the emotional and physical care of the patient. The problem illustrated in this case example is one that was related to us by a nurse in a geriatric setting. Caregiver support is defined as provision of the necessary information, advocacy, and support to facilitate primary patient care by people other than healthcare professionals (Craft & Willadsen, 1992). Again, the accompanying executive skills to operationalize the interventions are given.

Parent-Child System Problem: An elderly parent wants his or her adult children to visit more; the adult children do not enjoy visiting because their elderly parent is always complaining.

Domains of Family Functioning	Interventions: Encouraging family members to be caregivers and caregiver support
Cognitive and Behavioral	Teach adult children that their aging parent is having difficulty remembering their visits (short-term memory deficits), which is a common phenomenon of aging. Therefore, it is not useful to remind their aging parent of when they visited last.
Affective	Empathize with the aging parent, say that you understand that it must be lonely at times being a resident in a geriatric care center. The adult children would appreciate knowing that their parent is lonely so that they can respond appropriately. Therefore, advise the elderly parent to avoid complaining to the children that they do not visit enough, and instead, to tell them when they come that "Sometimes, I feel lonely here. I'm really glad you came to visit me."
Behavioral	Advise the adult children to stop giving excuses and explaining why they cannot come more often. Instead, obtain a guest book or calendar and write down each visit. Write down *who* visited and on *what* day, and perhaps any interesting news, so that the aging parent may read this between visits.

In each of the above examples, there are many other interventions and executive skills that could have been suggested. We believe very strongly that there is no one "right" intervention, only "useful" or "effective" interventions. How useful or effective an intervention is can only be evaluated after the intervention has been implemented. The element of time must be taken into account. With some interventions, the change or outcome may be noted immediately. However, it is more common that changes (outcomes) will not be noticed for a lengthy period of time. Most problems do not occur overnight, and the resolution of problems requires an appropriate length of time. Change can be observed, as Bateson (1979) states, as "difference which occurs across time" (p. 452).

CLINICAL CASE EXAMPLE 3

To appreciate that change is observed across time, we now offer two actual case examples of clinical work, from beginning to end, with the emphasis on the interventions that are used. A family was referred to one of our graduate nursing students with the presenting problems of enuresis and disciplinary problems at school with the eldest child, an 8-year-old boy. The family was composed of the father, age 28, self-employed; stepmother, age 21, homemaker; and two male children, ages 8 and 6. The couple had been married for about 1 year. The family was seen (as a whole family and in various subsystems) for a total of six sessions for 13 weeks from initial contact to termination.

A thorough family assessment (using the CFAM model) revealed the following problems:

Whole Family System Problem: Adjustment to being a blended family.

All family members were trying to adjust to a new family structure. After only being married a very short time, this stepmother found herself thrust into a parenting role when she and her husband became responsible for his two children, ages 6 and 4. The natural mother had deserted the children after living with them for 2 years in her home. The children had to adjust to a new set of parents, new surroundings, and no present contact with their natural mother.

Interventions. In the first session, the graduate student acknowledged that the problems the family was experiencing were a usual part of the adjustment of stepfamilies. The intervention of offering information/ opinions was directed at the cognitive domain of family functioning. This new information seemed to relieve the parents a great deal. Also, the student gave advice by encouraging the parents to allow the children to have contact with their biological mother if and when the biological mother once again sought them out. Initially, the parents were hesitant about this suggestion, but they later stated that they could see the importance of this for the children. The eldest child's problem of enuresis was conceptualized as a response to the adjustment to a stepfamily and the loss of his mother. This new opinion, also directed at the cognitive domain of family functioning, had a very positive effect on the family. The problem of enuresis dramatically improved over the course of treatment.

Parent-Child Subsystem Problem: Maladaptive interactional pattern between stepmother and eldest son (see circular pattern diagram below).

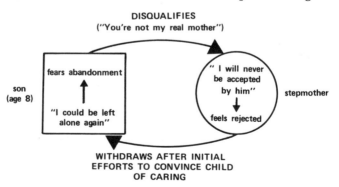

Due to the children's initial experience of the loss of their father (result of natural parents' divorce) and then literal abandonment by their biological mother, the children, particularly the eldest child, feared being abandoned again. Thus, the eldest child's effort to be reassured that he would not be abandoned again was to frequently tell his young stepmother that she was not his real mother. Initially, the stepmother would make efforts to reassure him but would eventually withdraw in frustration and feel rejected. This served as further fuel to maintain the maladaptive interactional pattern because the eldest child perceived this withdrawal as further evidence that he would be abandoned again. The vicious cycle was evident.

Interventions. The graduate nursing student encouraged the stepmother to stop withdrawing and to offer the child continual and sustained reassurance by stating, "I know I'm not your mother, but your father and I love and care for you and want to look after you. We will not leave you." This intervention of parent support and education was aimed at the behavioral, affective, and cognitive domains of family functioning. The behavioral task suggested to the stepmother proved to be quite successful. When the stepmother offered more reassurance to the boy, she reported that the boy ceased rejecting her. With decreased rejection, the stepmother was able to offer even more reassurance. Thus, a virtuous cycle began. The student also offered commendations of family strengths (intervention directed at the cognitive domain of family functioning) to the stepmother for her efforts to fulfill her role, as she was an exceptionally warm and caring young mother. The stepmother reported that she felt more relaxed in her parenting following this intervention.

Individual Problem: Eldest child's behavioral problems at school.

To assess this behavioral problem further, our graduate student met with the child's teacher at school and also discussed the problem twice with the teacher by phone. The stepmother was also present during the session at school.

Interventions. The main objective was to enhance the eldest child's self-esteem by focusing on his positive behavior. The teacher agreed to implement an intervention focused at the behavioral domain of family functioning: to acknowledge the child's positive behavior in front of his classmates in order to give him a different status than being the "clown of the class." It was also recommended to the stepmother that she minimize her contacts with the school and allow the teacher to assume more responsibility for the boy's behavior in class. Within a few weeks, the teacher reported a positive change in the child's behavior at school. The parents expressed great satisfaction over their child's improvement in school.

On termination with this family, the student recommended some readings on stepfamilies to the parents and also informed them of a "self-help group" for stepfamilies. These two interventions of bibliotherapy and providing information on community resources were targeted at all three domains of family functioning: cognitive, affective, and behavioral.

CLINCAL CASE EXAMPLE 4

A family was referred to one of our undergraduate students while the student had a community-health field placement, with the presenting problem being the social isolation and frequent physical complaints of a 78-year-old widowed mother. This senior lived in a government subsidized, one-bedroom apartment. She had six adult children (a son, age 51; a son, age 48; a daughter, age 44; a son, age 41; a son age 37; and a son, age 35) and 12 grandchildren. Five of the adult children were married, and all six children lived in the same city as their mother. The family was seen as a whole and in various subsystems for eight home visits over a period of 2 months.

Following a thorough family assessment (using the CFAM model) and individual assessment the following core problem was identified:

Whole Family System Problem: Mother's lack of social contact beyond immediate family.

It became apparent that this older woman was overly dependent on her adult children and, therefore, did not extend herself to be involved with her peers or in social activities appropriate to her age group. This resulted in frequent disagreements between the mother and the adult children over the frequency of visits with the mother. This was further exacerbated by the fact that the mother had no friends. After the death of her husband, about 10 years ago, she had lived intermittently with some of her adult children, but for the past 4 years had been living alone in her one-bedroom apartment. Presently, the youngest son visits the most and does his mother's grocery shopping.

Interventions. The student's first significant intervention was to broaden the context in order to expand her view and understanding of this family member's problem. Thus, the student initially interviewed the mother individually, then with her youngest son (the adult child who visited most frequently), and then the student took on the ambitious task of arranging an interview with the mother and her six adult children. This was a significant effort on the student's part to create a context for change. It had been agreed in the interview with the mother and her youngest son that the mother would contact the children. However, on follow-up by the student, it was learned that the mother had not called any of her children because she expected her youngest son to do it. This was further evidence of the mother's overdependence on her children. Because the youngest son was anxious to have a meeting with his mother and siblings, he had taken on the task of inviting all of his siblings to an interview with his mother and the student.

At the family interview, two of the adult children's spouses attended as well! Interestingly, the daughters-in-law were more vocal than their husbands and stated that they were very involved with their mother-in-law. In this large family interview, the issue of the mother's social isolation (apart from her family) was discussed. Through the process of circular questioning, the mother's and the adult children's expectations of contact were assessed. Initially, the student encouraged the family to explore alternative solutions to their mother's lack of social activities and a peer group. This intervention aimed at the behavioral domain of family functioning was met by a statement that they had no other ideas beyond what they had already tried. Therefore, the student offered some more specific interventions that might open solutions to the problem of the mother's social isolation. This important interview revealed that this older mother had always relied on her children for her main social interaction. The mother had never been a "joiner." In the past few years, she had even discontinued her attendance at church. Throughout her life she had had few close friends.

The assessment also revealed that collectively, the adult children had generally been supportive to their mother. Each week she had lunch with one or more of them. They included her in all special family occasions. However, the adult children always had to initiate contact. The children were genuinely concerned about their mother's loneliness and lack of additional social contact but had exhausted their ideas for changing the situation.

One of the first interventions the nursing student offered was directed at both the cognitive and behavioral domains of family functioning. The student offered information regarding community resources available to the older parent. Particularly, the student made the family aware of the Community Services Visitor Program. A decision was made that the mother would contact this program and the adult children would provide support in this effort. The mother also expressed interest in being involved in a choir again. The student offered to accompany her to a senior citizen's choir practice and introduce her to other participants.

The final major intervention discussed in that session was directed at the behavioral domain. The mother was asked if she would initiate contact with one of her adult children the next week. Following the contact, the adult child would ask the mother over for a visit as soon as possible. It has been our experience that the interest of family members in the senior's activities does much to increase the senior's motivation. It is important to emphasize that the older mother was involved in and receptive to these interventions.

The effect/outcome of these interventions was as follows:

1. The mother followed through on contacting the Community Services Visitor Program. The coordinator of the program contacted the mother and arranged for a regular visitor.
2. The student accompanied the mother to the senior citizen's choir. The older woman enjoyed the experience, and two of the other women in the choir telephoned afterward!
3. The mother took initiative to contact a couple of her adult children and

they in turn invited her over for a family visit, which she accepted. The children reported that they enjoyed their mother's calling them and this appeared to increase their own desire to have more frequent contact with her.

In future interviews, the student encouraged the mother to reconnect with her church. The student also solicited the support of the adult children in this endeavor by requesting that in their calls they take an interest and inquire about their mother's church and choir activities.

Because this older mother was accustomed to a good deal of family support, it was not appropriate to totally remove that support. However, physical instrumental support (doing things for the mother) could be reduced without the mother feeling abandoned. Verbal (emotional) support for the mother's attempts at independence was most appropriate. When the mother began to increase her social contacts and activities, there was also a decrease in the number of her nonspecific physical complaints.

The student concluded treatment with the older mother in a face-to-face interview. To involve the adult children in the termination process, the student sent a letter to each of the children. This letter, written by the student and her faculty supervisor, is printed verbatim below. It beautifully highlights the major interventions and again solicits further assistance from the adult children. Also, the student very nicely included some of the family strengths in the letter. Thus, the change process with this particular family will hopefully continue to evolve long after this nursing student's termination of the therapeutic relationship with this family.

Dear [real names omitted to preserve confidentiality]

I wish to thank you for your help and cooperation in my family assignment. I enjoyed meeting each of you and appreciated your individual input and assessment of your family. Your willingness to work together is certainly an excellent family strength.

I visited your mother on several occasions during my time with the Outreach Program. She continued to express her desire to be more socially independent. She has been able to make some increased community contact. She attended the choir and several of the choir ladies have called her to encourage her in continued participation. She met with the gentleman from the church and has spoken with his wife. The Coordinator of the Visitor Program visited and is arranging for a friend who will visit with your mother. Hopefully, they will develop some outside interests together. She has also been out to shop on her own on a few occasions.

I did contact Kerby Centre, as well as other seniors from Carter Place who go there, but was unable to find anyone going to the Wednesday lunch or any other suitable transportation. I have discussed this with your mother and she felt it might be something she could pursue on her own in the future.

Your mother expressed positive feelings about her attempts to be more socially active. However, she still looks to her children for her main support. At times I found she needed more encouragement not to overly worry about her health to the point that she thinks she is unable to participate in any activities. I believe that each of you may help your mother by encouraging her in this area. I might suggest that if she says that she is unwell that she see her doctor. If there is no serious problem, gentle support for her independent activities might be helpful. This may be somewhat difficult at first, but if you are able to present a united front to your mother and support each other in a mutual approach to her being more socially active, she may be more able to accomplish this.

I am very impressed with the cohesiveness of your family and the continued concern and support you show toward your mother. Thank you very much again for letting me work with you.

Yours truly,

Leslie Henderson
Undergraduate Nursing Student
Faculty of Nursing, University of Calgary

The therapeutic letter sent by the student is in and of itself an intervention. Also, several interventions, aimed at all three domains of family functioning, were embedded in the letter. Specifically, the student offered commendations and opinions directed at the cognitive domain of functioning; she invited the adult children to encourage their mother, which aimed at changes in the behavioral domain. By summarizing the clinical work with the family in the form of a therapeutic letter, the student intended to effect changes in both the affective and cognitive domains of family functioning. This very fine clinical work by an undergraduate student is an excellent example of how families can be effectively involved in healthcare when *family* assessment and intervention models are used with clear treatment goals and a student who is committed to improving family functioning through the development of her clinical skills.

HOW TO INTERVENE WITH COMMON FAMILY SITUATIONS NURSES ENCOUNTER

Having given four case examples illustrating the application of CFIM in clinical practice, we would now like to answer some questions we are asked frequently. These questions pertain to common family situations nurses frequently encounter.

QUESTION 1: HOW CAN NURSES HELP FAMILIES COPE WITH CHRONIC ILLNESS?

As a home care nurse, I have been working with a family in which the wife has multiple sclerosis. For several years they have coped fairly well. Within the past year, she has become progressively more physically and emotionally dependent. She insists that her husband stay at home every evening and that they spend every weekend together. He is anxious and told me he feels "trapped." He feels less and less able to help his wife. Yet he does not want to abandon her or to have her permanently hospitalized. How can I help this couple to cope more effectively with the wife's multiple sclerosis?

Discussion

The extent to which a person's illness affects the family often depends on the nature of the illness itself. If the illness is a prolonged and complicated one such as multiple sclerosis, it will most likely lead to differences in family relationships.

In working with a family in which one member has a chronic illness and requires additional care, the nurse should intervene and explore the family's cognition and beliefs about the illness. This intervention is aimed at the cognitive domain of family functioning. For example, the nurse in this instance may ask the husband and wife what they understand about multiple sclerosis, how the disease progresses, how long the periods of remission are, and so forth. In so doing, the nurse may be able to clear up misconceptions and provide further information.

Intervening with the Couple. When the nurse has established a baseline of the couple's understanding of multiple sclerosis, then the nurse can begin to explore their catastrophic expectations about the progression of the disease. Circular questions can be asked, such as:

To husband: What is the worst thing your wife fears as her multiple sclerosis progresses?

To wife: What is your husband's most pressing worry for the future?

These types of circular questions can be interchanged for husband and wife. Circular questions aimed at exploring one person's understanding of the other person's beliefs, expectations, and emotions can also be asked. These questions could also be asked directly to the patient or spouse. For example, the nurse could ask the patient, "What is the thing you fear most about your multiple sclerosis progressing?" By exploring the other person's understanding first, however, the nurse gains more information. If the husband answers that he thinks his wife fears most that he will have an affair, then this can be discussed during the interview. This two-step technique of asking the husband about the wife's expectations and then asking the wife directly about her own expectations is generally quite helpful in eliciting differences in beliefs.

After catastrophic expectations have been uncovered, they can realistically be discussed. When these fears of impending catastrophe remain hidden, they tend to impede problem-solving and promote isolation and maladaptive interaction patterns. In this case, if the wife fears that the husband will lose interest in her as her disease progresses, then this needs to be explored further. If the husband feels trapped and resentful about future care of his wife, then this too needs to be explored. Some questions that may guide the discussion include:

To wife: How do you show your feelings of fear? What do you do? What effect does this have on your husband? Is that the effect you would like it to have?

To husband: How do you deal with the extra demands of the illness? How do you show your feelings to your wife? What effect does this behavior seem to have on her?

These types of circular questions are aimed at increasing the family's understanding of the present situation. They provide a focus for the nurse to explore not only the family's cognition but also its underlying emotional responses. For example, the husband may feel resentful, anxious, and trapped and may be dealing with these feelings by isolating himself. The wife may be fearful and behave in a clutching, clingy fashion. Both of them may be unaware of the circular nature of the maladaptive pattern.

When the nurse has assisted the couple in recognizing the nature of their problem, then the nurse can help them explore alternative coping strategies leading to new solutions. For example, the nurse may stimulate the discussion by asking the following questions:

- How can you deal more realistically with the extra demands on both of you?
- What possibilities might work?
- What probably would never work?
- Who might be most upset if you were to, for example, invite a volunteer from the church in on Saturday to assist with the caretaking?

In summary, the main way the nurse can assist a family with a chronically ill member is to help them remove cognitive and affective blocks to problem-solving. If the husband is immobilized by guilt and a belief that he is losing his wife because of her illness and if the wife is immobilized by fear, then these blocks need to be gently dislodged to permit creative problem-solving to take place.

QUESTION 2: HOW CAN NURSES IMPROVE FAMILY VISITS WITH THE ELDERLY?

I work in an extended-care facility for the chronically ill. I have frequently noticed that when family members visit an elderly person they often find it difficult to communicate with that individual. One family found that their father was either sleeping, confused, or unresponsive whenever they would come to the hospital unit. They would then come to my office and talk with me. The family members complained that they could not talk with their relative. They made the trip to visit the patient; yet they ended up visiting with me. I often felt caught between the family and the patient. Do you have any suggestions as to how I can help family members to have a satisfying visit?

Discussion

It is well known that satisfaction with family relationships is very important to the elderly. There is a significant association between a positive elderly-parent–adult-child relationship and health and attitude toward aging factors (Watson, 1984). Satisfactory family relationships are the greatest single impact on life satisfaction for both men and women over age 65 (Medley, 1976).

The issue of a gap in communication between relatives and an elderly patient is a very critical topic not only for the family but also for the nursing staff. If an elderly person has a confidant, he or she is less likely to show mental impairment. Having someone to talk over problems with reduces the elderly person's preoccupation with future crisis. Many elders feel secure if they perceive their children as knowledgeable regarding their personal desires should a crisis occur.

In light of this, it is important for nurses to find ways to bring family members and elderly patients together. One suggestion is to set up an initial meeting with each side of the relationship, that is, the elder and other family members. A separate interview with the elder has the advantage that the nurse already knows the patient and can choose an optimal time to talk with him or her. The nurse can capitalize on the elder's alert moments. A separate interview with the family members affords an opportunity for the nurse to educate them about the process of aging.

Intervening with the Elderly Person. During the interview with the elderly person the nurse could:

- Ask which of the family members the elder would prefer to see most often.
- Find out how many people the elder prefers to visit at one time. For example, a son, daughter-in-law, and three grandchildren may be too overwhelming for the elder.
- Discuss with the elder and with the rest of the nursing staff what times of day the elder is most alert and responsive. In this way, visits may be able to be timed most appropriately.
- Ask where the elder feels most comfortable receiving visitors. (An Irish-American man may feel embarrassed to visit with his relatives in his bedroom, whereas a Latin-American man may enjoy the informality and intimacy.)
- Discuss how long the elder would like family members' visits to be.
- Ask if the elder would like to participate in any activities with the visitors. For example, a visit could be arranged in the coffee shop over lunch or dinner if this is suitable.
- Ask if there is anything the elder would like the family members to

bring from home but has been reluctant to ask for, like photographs or a special book.

Intervening with Family Members. During this session, the nurse could discuss with the family members the same issues discussed with the elderly patient. In this way, the relatives will have time to consider their desires as well as to speculate on the desires of the patient. The nurse also can offer them information to increase their understanding of the elderly.

Nurse: I know that you'd like to visit more with your father. Have you thought of how many people he feels comfortable visiting with at one time?

Son: Hmmm.

Nurse: The reason I raise this is that we know that sometimes the elderly have more difficulty listening to two things at once than do younger people. So, if three family members visit at once, your Dad may have trouble keeping track of the conversation. . . .

In addition to raising these issues, the nurse could discuss the importance of nonverbal communication. Many family members feel frustrated if they cannot talk with the elderly. But perhaps just sitting and touching the patient's hand is comforting. Sitting and listening to a favorite piece of music (played on a portable tape recorder) can also be a satisfying visit for both parties.

Intervening with the Elderly Patient and the Family Together. After discussing these issues separately with the patient and the family, the nurse could then set up a joint interview for the next visit. A photograph of the persons who are coming to visit could be shown to the patient on the morning of the visit, and the staff could refer to the upcoming meeting. At this interview, the nurse should raise the same issues as were brought up in the previous sessions and stimulate discussion between the family members and the elderly person. The nurse can act as a coach for the elderly person if the elder forgets some of the issues raised in the individual sessions. A visiting plan could then be devised and tried for a month. During this time, the patient and the family would meet together without the nurse being present. After the trial period, the nurse could join the elderly patient and family in a meeting to evaluate the visits and discuss any needed modifications.

Basically, what the nurse needs to do is to detriangulate herself from the situation. The nurse initially functioned as a go-between for the family and the patient. The nurse's task was to foster direct and improved communication during visits. If, however, the nurse were to continue in the role of go-between, then it is unlikely that the family-patient relationship would progress. Rather, both the family and the patient would probably come to rely too heavily on the nurse's presence during the visits. Thus, the nurse might inadvertently foster *indirect* communication. We recommend that after having initial, separate meetings with the patient and the family the nurse should encourage joint meetings. If at a future date, a meeting with the relatives seems indicated (e.g., because of change in the elderly person's status), then the nurse should initiate such a session instead of having the family members revert back to dropping in to visit with the nurse.

QUESTION 3: HOW CAN NURSES ASSIST SINGLE-PARENT FAMILIES WHO ARE EXPERIENCING DIFFICULTIES?

In my community district there are many single-parent families. Most of these families are young women in their mid-20's who have at least two toddlers or preschoolers. Many of them have recently been divorced. They are generally overwhelmed at being on their own and have few support systems. They often look to me (and to other nurses in our unit) for support. One mother called last week and said, "I have no one to talk with and I feel I am drowning with all these problems." How can I help these women without taking sides regarding the issues in their divorce and without becoming overinvolved?

Discussion

Working with single-parent families presents a challenge to nurses in a variety of healthcare settings. Glick (1989) found that single-parents constituted 11 percent of all families in the United States in 1988, with about 1 out of every 7 of these families being maintained by the father, as compared with 1 out of every 10 in 1960. It is not surprising, therefore, that CHNs who deal with preschoolers are becoming increasingly involved with single-parent families.

Severe emotional distress is sometimes prevalent in the lives of single-parent adults in the first year following divorce. Their self-esteem is decreased, their anxiety is increased, and they have feelings of external control over their lives (Heatherington, Cox, & Cox, 1980). With regard to the instrumental aspects of daily living, single parents face role adjustments, especially in the areas of home management and child care. Hill (1986) reports that single-parent families must accomplish most of the same developmental tasks as do two-parent families but without all the resources. They frequently experience a lack of social support during the early aftermath of divorce.

Children are also affected emotionally by their parents' decision to separate. Based on their research, Wallerstein and Kelly (1980) have delineated some different outcomes for children of various ages and developmental stages in the first year after divorce. They found that many youngsters typically reacted with denial and often assumed that they "caused the divorce." Young preschoolers (age $2^{1}/_{2}$ to $3^{1}/_{2}$) frequently experience intense regression in cognition, behavior, and self-control, while older preschoolers (age $3^{3}/_{4}$ to $4^{3}/_{4}$) tend to demonstrate self-blame, diminished self-esteem, and disruptions in their sense of order and predictability. Five-year-olds have been shown to respond with anxiety, sadness, irritability, and temper tantrums. Young school-age children (age 6 to 8) demonstrate sadness and fear, while older children (age 9 to 12) express anger, especially at the noncustodial parent. School-aged children (age 6 to 12) experience divided loyalties and often are thrust into alignments with one parent against the other. Thirteen- to 18-year-olds experience a profound sense of loss and anger, which may impede their progression through adolescence.

Intervening with the Family. In light of these typical (although transitory) reactions to marital dissolution, it is not surprising that many single parents seek assistance from either professionals or self-help groups in the first year following divorce. Nurses can often assist both the parent and the children in dealing with these issues during the stressful immediate postdivorce period.

First, nurses can *provide the parent with information about normal growth and development and the predictable effects of divorce on children.* This is especially important for single-parent fathers, who often lack knowledge about what constitutes normalcy. Single-parent mothers who are thrust into the workforce may not have sufficient opportunity to keep track of their child's developmental milestones. Families also appreciate knowing that there are stages to the divorce process. Following the initial crisis period, the majority of adults are able to acknowledge the beneficial effects of divorce and readjust.

Second, during the crisis of divorce, *single parents need to learn how to help their children cope effectively.* During the immediate postdivorce period, single parents may have great difficulty attending to their children's needs; for example, they may avoid telling the children about the divorce or assuring them of continued care, may have less face-to-face contact with them, and often are less consistent in their discipline than are two-parent households (Heatherington, Cox, & Cox, 1980). Yet, youngsters need sufficient opportunity at this critical time to express their concerns. The parent needs to recognize that divorce is indeed a family crisis. This is difficult because many parents feel uncomfortable dealing with their children's emotional upsets. Keshet and Rosenthal (1980) found that 44 percent of single-parent fathers requested help from other people to deal with their children's feelings. Thus, the nurse can help these families by modeling how to talk with children about the impact of divorce. In addition, the nurse can focus on the sibling subsystem, as it is the subsystem that usually remains intact during the process of family reorganization. Schibuk (1989) suggests that sibling therapy can be effective, as children are the "unit of continuity" (p. 226).

A third way in which nurses can be useful to single parents is to *provide information about and normalize stress.* Single parents should know about the stresses they can expect in their own lives. These can be categorized into instrumental stress and personal, emotional stress. In areas of instrumental stress, single parents report great difficulty coping with day-care facilities and transportation of children, use of babysitters, and other support systems. The nurse can discuss the available facilities in the community, means of accessing them, financial arrangements, and so forth. In the area of emotional stress, low self-esteem, loneliness, depression, feelings of helplessness, and high anxiety appear to be characteristic of both men and women in the immediate postdivorce period. In working with these families, the nurse is advised to maintain as neutral an attitude as possible about the divorce and to establish short-term goals. The nurse may be a tremendous help in aiding the parent to sort out feelings of confusion and disappointment about the loss of the marital relationship. The nurse can also encourage the parent to continue to deal with unfinished emotional business.

Finally, nurses can intervene with single parents by *encouraging them to mobilize a personal support system.* This support system will further help them deal with their emotional and instrumental stress over the long term. For example, the nurse can discuss the importance and benefit of a support network with the mother at the time of her first visit. The nurse can ask the mother to invite a friend to the next interview. In this way, the nurse, the patient, and the friend will meet to discuss issues. Gradually, the nurse can remove herself as a source of support, and the patient will have her own natural support network. This will help the nurse to avoid becoming the primary support system for the mother. Just as it is important for a child in a single-parent household to avoid becoming a surrogate spouse, so too it is important for the nurse to avoid assuming this role.

Nurses can also encourage single parents to form groups that can be of both emotional and instrumental help to themselves. Many communities have support organizations and courses for single parents. The nurse should be familiar with these courses and organizations to be able to promote their use by single-parent families in need of such external support.

CONCLUSIONS

Interventions can be straightforward and simple or as innovative and dramatic as the nurse deems necessary for the health problem(s) presented. Ell and Northen (1990) convincingly write and support this statement with abundant research documentation that "interventions intended to promote health and prevent illness should be based on the assumption that individual health behaviors are strongly influenced by those around us, and that family general well-being can promote the physical health of its members" (p. 79). Any interventions should be directed toward the goals of treatment collaboratively generated by the nurse *and* the family. As nurses learn to actively engage, thoroughly assess, and clearly identify problems, and to set treatment goals and solutions, the conceptualizing, choosing, and implementing of specific interventions with each family becomes more rewarding and more effective. The ultimate goal, of course, is to assist family members to discover new solutions to their problems through the interventions that are offered.

REFERENCES

Bateson, G. (1979). *Steps to an ecology of mind.* New York: Ballatine Books.

Craft, M. J., & Willadsen, J. A. (1992). Interventions related to family. *Nursing Clinics of North America, 27*(2), 517–540.

de Shazer, S. (1988). Clues: *Investigating solutions in brief therapy.* New York: W. W. Norton.

Duhamel, F. (1987). Assessing families of adolescents with Crohn's disease. In L. M. Wright & M. Leahey (Eds.), *Families and chronic illness* (pp 168–185). Springhouse, PA: Springhouse.

Ell, K. & Northen, H. (1990). *Families and health care.* New York: Aldine de Gruyter.

Fleuridas, C., Nelson, T., & Rosenthal, D. (1986). The evolution of circular questions: Training family therapists. *Journal of Marital and Family Therapy, 12*(2), 113–127.

Glick, P. C. (1989). The family life cycle and social change. *Family Relations, 38,* 123–129.

Heatherington, E., Cox., M., & Cox, R. (1980). The aftermath of divorce. In P. Mussen, J. Conger, & J. Kagan (Eds.), *Readings in child and adolescent psychology* (pp. 163–177). New York: Harper & Row.

Hill, R. (1986). Life cycle stages for types of single-parent families: Of family development theory. *Family Relations, 35,* 19–29.

Imber-Black, E., Roberts, J., & Whiting, R. (Eds.). (1988). *Rituals in families and family therapy.* New York: W. W. Norton.

Jessee, E. H., Jurkovic, G. J., Wilkie, J., & Chiglinski, M. (1982). Positive reframing with children: Conceptual and clinical considerations. *American Journal of Orthopsychiatry, 52,* 314–322.

Keshet, H., & Rosenthal, K. (1980). Single-parent fathers: A new study. In P. Mussen, J. Conger, & J. Kagan (Eds.), *Readings in child and adolescent psychology* (pp. 184–188). New York: Harper & Row.

Leahey, M., & Wright, L. M. (1987). Families and chronic illness: Assumptions, assessment, and intervention. In L. M. Wright & M. Leahey (Eds.), *Families and chronic illness* (pp. 55–76). Springhouse, PA: Springhouse.

Lipchik, E., & de Shazer, S. (1986). The purposeful interview. *Journal of Strategic and Systemic Therapies, 5,* 88–99.

Loos, F., & Bell, J. M. (1990). Circular questions: A family interviewing strategy. *Dimensions of Critical Care Nursing, 9*(1), 46–53.

Maturana, H., & Varela, F. (1992). *The tree of knowledge: The biological roots of human understanding.* Boston: Shambhala.

McElheran, N., & Harper-Jaques, S. (1994). Commendations: A resource intervention for clinical practice. *Clinical Nurse Specialist.*

Medley, M. (1976). Satisfaction with life among persons sixty-five years and older. *Journal of Gerontology, 31,* 448–455.

Mischke-Berkey, K., Warner, P., & Hanson, S. (1989). Family health assessment and intervention. In P. J. Bomar (Ed.), *Nurses and family health promotion: Concepts, assessment and intervention* (pp. 115–154). Baltimore: Williams & Wilkins.

Roberts, J. (1988). Setting the frame: Definition, functions, and typology of rituals. In E. Imber-Black, J. Roberts, & R. Whiting (Eds.), *Rituals in families and family therapy* (pp. 3–46). New York: W. W. Norton.

Schibuk, M. (1989). Treating the sibling subsystem: An adjunct of divorce therapy. *American Journal of Orthopsychiatry, 59*(2), 226–237.

Selvini-Palazzoli, M., Boscolo, L., Cecchin, G., & Prata, G. (1978). A ritualized prescription in family therapy: Odd days and even days. *Journal of Marriage and Family Counseling, 4*(3), 3–9.

Selvini-Palazzoli, M., Boscolo, L., Cecchin, G., & Prata, G. (1980). Hypothesizing—circularity–neutrality: Three guidelines for the conductor of the session. *Family Process, 19*(3), 3–12.

Thorne, S., & Robinson, C. (1989). Guarded alliance: Health-care relationships in chronic illness. *Image, 21(3),* 153–157.

Tomm, K. (1984). One perspective on the Milan systemic approach: 2. Description of session format, interviewing style and interventions. *Journal of Marital and Family Therapy, 10*(3), 253–271.

Tomm, K. (1985). Circular interviewing: A multifaceted clinical tool. In D. Campbell, & R. Draper (Eds.), *Applications of systemic family therapy: The Milan approach* (pp. 33–45). London: Grune & Stratton.

Tomm, K. (1987). Interventive interviewing: 2. Reflexive questioning as a means to enable self-healing. *Family Process, 26,* 167–183.

Tomm, K. (1988). Interventive interviewing: 3. Intending to ask lineal, circular, strategic or reflexive questions? *Family Process, 27,* 1–15.

Tomm, K. (1989). Externalizing the problem and internalizing personal agency. *Journal of Strategic and Systemic Therapies, 1(1),* 54–59.

Wallerstein, J., & Kelly, J. (1980). *Surviving the breakup: How children and parents cope with divorce.* New York: Basic Books.

Watson, W. L. (1984). *The effect of a psychoeducational program on adult daughters and their aging parents.* Unpublished doctoral dissertation, University of Calgary, Alberta.

Watson, W. L. (Producer). (1988a.) *A family with chronic illness: A "tough" family copes well* [Videotape]. Calgary, Alberta: University of Calgary.

Watson, W. L. (Producer). (1988b). *Aging families and Alzheimer's disease* [Videotape]. Calgary, Alberta: University of Calgary.

Watson, W. L. (Producer). (1988c). *Fundamentals of family systems nursing* [Videotape]. Calgary, Alberta: University of Calgary.

Watson, W. L. (Producer). (1989a). *Families and psychosocial problems* [Videotape]. Calgary, Alberta: University of Calgary.

Watson, W. L. (Producer). (1989b). *Family systems interventions* [Videotape]. Calgary, Alberta: University of Calgary.

Watson, W. (1992). Family therapy. In G. M. Bulechek & J. C. McCloskey (Eds.), *Nursing interventions: Essential nursing treatments* (pp. 379–391). Philadelphia: W. B. Saunders.

Watson, W. L., & Nanchoff-Glatt, M. (1990). A family systems nursing approach to premenstrual syndrome. *Clinical Nurse Specialist, 4*(1) 3–9.

Watzlawick, P., Weakland, J., & Fisch, R. (1974). *Change: Principles of problem formulation and problem resolution.* New York: W. W. Norton.

White M. (1984). Psuodo-encopresis: From avalanche to victory, from vicious to virtuous circles. *Family Systems Medicine, 2,* 150–160.

White, M. (1986). Negative explanation, restraint and double description: A template for family therapy. *Family Process, 25,* 160–184.

White M. (1988). The process of questioning: A therapy of literary merit. *Dulwich Centre Newsletter,* 8–14.

White, M. (1988–1989). The externalizing of the problem and the re-authoring of lives and relationships. *Dulwich Centre Newsletter,* 3–21.

White, M., & Epston, M. (1989). *Literate means to therapeutic ends.* Adelaide, Australia: Dulwich Centre Publications.

Wright, L. M., & Leahey, M. (1987). Families and life-threatening illness: Assumptions, assessment, and intervention. In M. Leahey & L. M. Wright (Eds.), *Families and life-threatening illness* (pp. 45–58). Springhouse, PA: Springhouse.

Wright, L. M., & Levac, A. M. (1992). The non-existence of non-compliant families: The influence of Humberto Maturana. *Journal of Advanced Nursing, 17,* 913–917.

Wright, L. M., & Park Dorsay, J. (1989). A case of Marilynitis or a Marilyn Monroe infection. Adelaide, Australia: *Dulwich Centre Newsletter,* 7–9.

Wright, L. M., & Simpson, P. (1991). A systemic belief approach to epileptic seizures: A case of being spellbound. *Contemporary Family Therapy: An International Journal, 13*(2), 165–180.

CHAPTER 5

FAMILY INTERVIEWING: COMPETENCIES AND SKILLS

When the nurse has a clear conceptual framework for assessing and intervening with families, she can then begin to consider the competencies and skills needed for family interviews. The types of skills identified as necessary by various authors on family work reflect each author's particular theoretical orientation and preference as to how to approach and resolve problems. Therefore, the skills that are delineated in this chapter are based on *our* theoretical foundation of the systems, cybernetic, communication, and change theories that inform CFAM and CFIM. We favor a problem/solution-focused and time-limited approach. We emphasize that families possess the ability to solve their own problems, and that our task as nurses is to facilitate and assist them to find their own solutions. We do not propose that we know what is "best" for families. However, to be involved in helping families change requires that nurses possess certain essential competencies and skills.

In the previous chapters we discussed the knowledge base that is necessary for beginning practice with families in order to competently assess and intervene with them. This chapter focuses on the specific beginning-level skills necessary for family interviewing. We concur with the Alberta Association of Registered Nurses' (AARN, 1991) Nursing Practice Standards and Competencies for Nurses, which defines competencies as "the ability to demonstrate the requisite knowledge, skills and attitudes of nurses beginning to practice" (p. 2). The AARN (1991) specifically describes the importance of reciprocal/interactional knowledge of families by stating that one of the knowledge competencies required of the nurse is that she "recognizes the influence of family structure and functioning on the patient/client's health status and the influence of health status on family functioning" (p. 3).

In the past 20 years, the explosion of literature on family work suggests and implies a myriad of skills that can be employed when working with families (Allred & Kersey, 1977; Falicov, Constantine, & Breunlin, 1981; Haley, 1987; Liddle, 1991; Tomm & Wright, 1979; Watson, 1992). Cleghorn and Levin (1973), however, point out that simply stating general skills such as "the student must be able to label interactions accurately" says nothing about how that skill can be achieved. Figley and Nelson (1989) conducted a survey of educators and trainers of family therapists to identify the most important skills for beginners. The five most important skills identified were (1) basic interviewing skills, (2) establishing rapport, (3) giving credit for positive changes, (4) being able to distinguish content from process, and (5) setting reachable goals. Another very interesting finding of this study was that 31 percent of their top 100 generic skills referred to personal traits.

Through the use of specific learning objectives, the mystery of what a family interviewer actually does is removed. Thus, the learning objectives or skills become the "map of the interview," just as the Calgary Family Assessment Model (CFAM) serves as the "map of the family." Therefore, the skills described in this chapter are approach-specific skills that emerge out of the application of CFAM and CFIM. These skills become the nurse behaviors that are unique to working with families. Of course, each nurse brings her own unique genetic makeup and history of interactions, which personalize the application of these skills.

STAGES OF FAMILY INTERVIEWS

Four major stages of family interviewing can be identified within the context of a therapeutic conversation between a nurse and a family. These are engagement, assessment, intervention, and termination. These stages tend to follow in a logical sequence both during the course of a given interview and during the overall course of contact. For example, a nurse engages family members during each interview and terminates with them at the end of each interview, as well as at the beginning and end of the entire contact.

Engagement refers to the first stage, in which the nurse exercises skills that will establish and maintain a therapeutic relationship with the family. Selvini-Palazzoli, Boscolo, Cecchin, and Prata (1980) suggest that the interviewer should be allied with everyone and no one at the same time. They refer to this process as *neutrality.* It has also been called *curiosity* (Cecchin, 1987). Those factors that appear to inhibit engagement by the family interviewer are confrontation and interpretation too early in treatment (Gurman & Kniskern, 1981). Further ideas and suggestions for the engagement stage are given in Chapters 6 and 7.

Assessment, the second stage, includes the substages of problem exploration and identification, plus delineation of a strengths and problem list. Beginning nurse interviewers generally lack a clear stepwise rationale to guide the collecting and processing of data during an interview. Thus, beginners often spend an inordinate amount of time collecting vast amounts of information. Frequently, this information is tangential to the presenting problem and is not usable. Alternatively, beginners sometimes rush into inappropriate treatment because they are without a clear formulation of the presenting problem. It is better, however, for beginners to err on the side of taking longer than usual to complete the initial assessment than to rush to the intervention stage too prematurely. It needs to be noted that assessment in family work is an ongoing process. Thus, the strengths and problems list may change over time as the nurse's conceptual understanding of the family becomes more systemic. Ideas for what to assess and how to integrate and document the information are available in Chapters 3 and 8, respectively.

The *intervention,* or third stage, is really the core of clinical work with families. It involves providing a context in which the family may make small or significant changes. There are numerous ways in which to intervene, and treatment plans should be tailored to each family. The Calgary Family Intervention Model (Chapter 4) provides a specific "map for the nurse" and offers examples of specific interventions that can be utilized by nurses.

Termination, the last stage, refers to the process of relinquishing the therapeutic relationship between the nurse and the family in a manner that allows the family not only to maintain but to continue constructive changes. Therapeutic termination encourages family members in their ability to solve problems in the future. Specific ideas for therapeutic termination are described in Chapter 9.

TYPES OF SKILLS

Within each stage of family interviewing there are three types of skills: perceptual, conceptual, and executive (Cleghorn & Levin, 1973). The identification and categorization of these three sets of skills by Cleghorn and Levin (1973) is considered to be a seminal contribution (Liddle, 1991). These authors were the first to offer a systematic way to think about training family therapists and provided "a conceptual scaffolding" (Liddle, 1991, p. 640). Tomm and Wright (1979) used the perceptual, conceptual, and executive skills model as a guide for their comprehensive outline, which offered examples of therapist functions, competencies, and skills in each category over the course of family therapy. In our text, we have kept Wright's previous experience of identifying particular perceptual, conceptual, and executive skills across the four stages of family interviews. However, we have adapted the perceptual, conceptual, and executive skills to be congruent with nurses who are beginning to practice with families. The skills that we have identified fit within the context of our particular models, namely, CFAM and CFIM. Perceptual and conceptual skills are paired because what is perceived is so intimately interrelated with what is thought. It is often difficult to separate the perceptual from the conceptual component. These perceptual/conceptual skills are then matched with executive skills.

Perceptual skills refer to the nurse's ability to make pertinent and accurate observations. However, there is a major shift from the perceptual skills required in individual interviewing to those required in family interviewing. Goren (1979) points out this shift by stating that the interviewer's "initial energies are directed at observing the family system in action, and abstracting from that observation the repetitive patterns of interactions among family members" (p. 458).

Conceptual skills involve the ability to give meaning to observations. They also involve the ability to formulate one's observations of the family as a whole, as a system. We are always cognizant that the meanings derived from observations are not necessarily true but represent one nurse's effort to make sense of her observations.

Janzen (1980) emphasizes that the student entering nursing has intuitive *perceptual/conceptual skills* that have been learned in other roles in previous life experiences. Many of the skills, however, are out of the student's awareness. The nurse needs to develop an overt awareness of the perceptual process. The perceptual/conceptual skills form the basis for the executive skills.

Executive skills are the therapeutic interventions that the nurse actually carries out in an interview. These skills or therapeutic interventions receive responses from family members and form the basis for the nurse's further observations and conceptualizations. As can be readily seen, the interview process is a circular phenomenon between the nurse and family.

DEVELOPMENT OF SKILLS

In the education of nurses regarding the nursing of families, emphasis should be placed first on the development of perceptual/conceptual skills. This can be accomplished by several methods. Lectures and readings are helpful. However, observation and videotapes of family interviews are a better way to increase perceptual and conceptual skill accuracy. When a nurse is unable to perform a specific executive skill, it is useful to find out whether the interviewer has developed a perceptual/conceptual base for that particular skill. This is the value of matching these skills in pairs.

Two surveys of nursing programs, one in Canada (Wright & Bell, 1989) and the other in the United States (Hanson & Heims, 1992), are an important beginning evaluation of our efforts as nurse educators to develop family interviewing skills. Both studies found that family assessment is generally well taught at the baccalaureate level but that family intervention skills at both the undergraduate and graduate levels are sadly lacking. Of particular interest was the minimal provision of live supervised clinical practice with families, particularly at the graduate level (Wright & Bell, 1989). Case discussion and process recording were reported as the predominant method of supervision. To develop and achieve therapeutic competence in nursing practice with families, it is essential that live supervision be provided (Wright, 1994).

The specific skills for interviewing families are listed in logical sequence. However, this does not mean that during the course of an actual interview, the nurse must follow this outline rigidly. The nurse needs a "map of interviewing skills" that allows for considerable flexibility in application.

FAMILY INTERVIEWING SKILLS FOR NURSES

Stage 1: Engagement

Perceptual/Conceptual Skills | Executive Skills

1. **Recognize that an individual family member is best understood in the context of the family.**
That is, no individual exists in isolation.

1. **Invite all family members who are concerned/involved with the problem to attend the first interview.**
For example, grandparents or other relatives or friends living outside of the home should also be invited to attend if they are involved in the problem.

2. **Appreciate that initial efforts to involve both spouses/ parents enables, from the onset, a more holistic view of the family and increases engagement.**
That is, fathers should definitely be involved for effective family work. Family therapy research (Gurman & Kniskern, 1981) indicates a much better outcome when fathers are present.

2. **Employ all efforts to initially involve both spouses/parents in initial sessions.**

3. **Recognize that providing a clear structure to the interview reduces anxiety and increases engagement.**
That is, there is generally anxiety related to the uncertainty of being in a new setting and of not knowing how to behave in the situation.

3. **Explain to family members the purpose, length, and structure of the interview and ask if they have any questions relating to the interview.**
For example, "I thought we could spend about 25 minutes together discussing the problems that you are concerned about in the family."

4. **Recognize that initially members are most comfortable talking about the structural aspects of the family.**
That is, note nonverbal cues indicating level of comfort, such as taking coat off, adequate versus minimal time spent talking, and participating in versus ignoring conversation.

4. **Ask *each* family member to relate information with regard to name, age, work or school, years married, and so forth.**
For example, identity yourself directly by giving your name and either shaking hands or making some physical contact (e.g., touching a child's head).

Stage 2: Assessment

Perceptual/Conceptual Skills

Executive Skills

1. **Realize the importance of having a conceptual assessment map to understand family dynamics.**
That is, a conceptual assessment map provides the nurse with several possible courses for focused exploration.

1. **Explore the components of the structural, developmental, and functional aspects of CFAM to assess strengths and problem areas.**
All components of CFAM need not be explored if they are not relevant to the present issues.

2. **Realize the importance of beginning a family assessment by obtaining a detailed description and history of the presenting problem.**
That is, because the presenting problem usually serves as an entry point to understanding how the family functions, it is worthwhile to be thorough in collecting data with regard to it.

2. **Ask each family member, including the children, to share his or her knowledge and understanding of the presenting problem.**
For example, ask the father, "How do you see the problem?" or ask the whole family, "What is the main problem that each of you would like to see changed?"

3. **Realize that the presenting problem is often related to other problems in the family.**
That is, a child's temper tantrums may be related to the parents' marital conflict (e.g., the child may be triangulated into the marital conflict).

3. **Explore with the family if there are other problems/concerns connected to the presenting problem(s).**
For example, "We've been talking for some time about the problem of Danielle's temper tantrums. I'm wondering if there are any other problems the family is concerned about at present."

4. Realize that eliciting differences generates more specific information for family assessment.
That is:
(a) Clarification of differences between individuals is a significant source of information about *family functioning.*

(b) Clarification of differences between relationships is a significant source of information about *family structure/alliances.*
(c) Clarification of differences in family members or in relationships at various points in time is a significant source of information about *family development.*

5. Use the information obtained from the family assessment to begin formulating hypotheses in the form of a strengths/ problems list.
That is, structural, developmental, and functional strengths/problems may be present at various systems levels. For example, whole family system problems:
(a) Structural: adjusting to new family form of single-parent family.
(b) Developmental: family in life cycle stage of children leaving home.
(c) Functional: Family belief, "Father would be displeased with us for still crying about his death."

4. Inquire about differences between individuals, between relationships, and between various points in time.
For example:
(a) To explore differences between individuals, ask the child: "What is expected of you before you go to bed at night?" and then ask, "Who is the best, Mother or Father, at getting you to do those things in the evening?"

(b) To explore differences between relationships ask: "Do Father and Mark fight more or less than Father and Hannah?"
(c) To explore differences before or after important points in time ask: "Do you worry more, less, or the same about your husband's health since his heart attack?"

5. Obtain verification of nurse's understanding of strengths/ problems by listing them to the family and eventually recording them.
For example: "We've identified that being a new single parent and also having to cope with your children leaving home are your two major concerns. We've also discussed that your family is very well-liked in the community."

6. **Assess whether any of the identified problems are beyond the scope of the nurse's competence.**

   That is, it is appropriate to consider referral when medical symptoms have not been fully assessed or long-standing emotional or behavioral problems exist.

6. **Tell the family whether or not you will continue to work with them on problems. (If a decision is made to refer them to another professional, proceed to Stage 4A: Termination.)**

   For example, tell the family: "Now that I have a more complete understanding of your concerns, I think it necessary to have your son's headaches checked out medically. I would like to refer you to a pediatrician."

7. **Recognize that a more extensive inquiry into the most pressing problems is necessary before intervention plans can be implemented.**

   That is, initially families are usually most concerned with the presenting problem.

7. **Seek the family's opinion of which issue they perceive as most important and explore it in depth. If the family cannot agree, then discuss the lack of consensus.**

   For example, ask: "About which of the problems we have discussed today are you most concerned?"

8. **Recognize that the assessment is complete when sufficient information has been obtained to formulate a treatment plan.**

   That is, nurses sometimes rush into inappropriate treatment because they are without a clear understanding of the presenting problem or other significant related problems.

8. **State your integrated understanding of problem(s) to family and obtain their commitment to work on a specific problem.**

   For example, "Since the family agrees that Jeff's acting out is connected to the arguing between the parents, I would like to suggest that we focus on this problem for three interviews. Would you be willing?"

Stage 3: Intervention

Perceptual/Conceptual Skills

Executive Skills

1. **Recognize that family systems are goal-directed and possess problem-solving abilities.**

1. **Encourage family members to explore possible solutions to problems.**

That is, a belief that families not only possess the capability to change but also can identify and implement solutions of how to change helps the nurse to avoid becoming overcontrolling or overresponsible.

2. **Recognize that interventions are focused on the cognitive, affective, and/or behavioral domains of functioning in families, as described in the CFIM.**
That is, it is not always necessary or even efficient to target interventions at all *three* domains of functioning simultaneously.

3. **Recognize that lack of information of an educational nature can inhibit the family's problem-solving abilities.**
That is, often with additional information, families will be able to provide their own creative and unique solutions to problems.

4. **Recognize that persistent and intense emotions can often block the family's problem-solving abilities.**
That is, families who predominantly experience emotions such as sadness or anger are often unable to deal with problems until the emotional block is removed.

For example, "Susan, you've mentioned that your mother is too critical of herself. Do you have any ideas of what she could do to feel better about herself as a mother with a chronic illness?"

2. **Plan interventions to target any one or all three of the domains of functioning described in the CFIM.**
For example,
   (a) Cognitive: invite the family to think differently.
   (b) Affective: encourage different affective expression.
   (c) Behavioral: ask the family to perform new tasks either within or outside of the interview.

3. **Provide information to the family that will enhance its knowledge and facilitate further problem-solving.**
For example, the nurse can provide information about the normal reactions of a 3-year-old to a new baby, or about the aging process of an older adult. This type of intervention targets the family's cognitive domain of functioning.

4. **Validate family members' emotional responses, when appropriate.**
For example, suppression of grief over the loss of a family member may only need confirmation of the normal grieving process to free family members to work through their bereavement. This type of intervention targets the family's affective domain of functioning.

5. **Recognize that suggesting specific tasks can often provide a new way for family members to behave in relation to one another that will improve problem-solving abilities.**
That is, some tasks can serve to begin changes in the structure of the family and/or family rules.

5. **Assign tasks aimed at improving family functioning.**
That is, suggest the father and son spend one evening a week together in a common activity; suggest to the mother and father that one parent discipline the children on odd days and the other on even days. This type of intervention targets the family's behavioral domain of functioning.

Stage 4: Termination

Perceptual/Conceptual Skills

Executive Skills

A. If consultation or referral is necessary:

1. **Recognize that families appreciate additional professional resources when problems are quite complex.**
That is, nurses cannot be expected to be experts in all areas.

1. **Refer individuals and/or family members for consultation or ongoing treatment.**
For example, "I feel that your family needs professional input beyond what I can offer for Guillermo's learning disability problems. So I would like to refer you to the learning center in the city. They have more expertise in dealing with these types of problems."

B. If family interviewing with nurse continues:

1. **Recognize the importance of evaluating the family interviews at regular intervals.**
That is, evaluating the progress of family interviews leads to more focused and purposeful time spent with the family.

1. **Obtain feedback from family members about the present status of their problems and initiate termination when the contracted problems have been resolved or sufficient progress has been made.**
For example, it is not necessary to send families away problem-free but rather to have increased their ability and confidence to solve problems.

2. Recognize when dependency on the nurse inadvertently may have been encouraged. That is, many interviews over a prolonged period of time foster excessive dependency.

2. Mobilize other supports for the family if necessary, and begin to initiate termination by decreasing the frequency of sessions. For example, nurses can inadvertently provide "paid friendship," with mothers in particular, unless they mobilize other supports, such as husband, friends, or relatives.

3. Recognize family members' constructive efforts to solve problems.

3. Summarize positive efforts of family members to resolve problems whether or not significant improvement has occurred.

4. Recognize that backup support by professional resources is appreciated by individuals and families in times of stress.

4. End the family interviews with a face-to-face discussion when possible. Extend an invitation for further family interviews if appropriate, should problems recur.

PERCEPTIONS OF SKILL ATTAINMENT

How competent a nurse is when working with a particular family will have a direct relationship to the success of treatment. The Family Nursing Unit, University of Calgary, has found it useful to conduct a follow-up evaluation of the perceptions of Master of Nursing (MN) students regarding their attainment of clinical skills (Wright, Watson, & Bell, 1990). One year after graduation, each student is mailed a questionnaire developed for the study. The results to date (n = 32) suggest that family systems nursing skills can be acquired with supervision and maintained in clinical practice, regardless of the employment opportunities for direct, clinical contact with families. The most surprising finding has been the graduates' reports of a dramatic conceptual shift from a linear perspective to a more systemic "world view." The concepts identified as having the most impact on graduates' thinking are circularity and systems theory concepts, understanding the individual in the context of the family, the use of circular questions as interventions, and the reciprocal influence of illness and family functioning. Wright, Watson, and Bell (1990) suggest that the family, as the system of focus, becomes a vehicle for learning systemic concepts and skills that the MN graduates are then able to extrapolate to a variety of other settings and situations.

CONCLUSIONS

These family interviewing skills function as a guide for the nurse when working with a family. Thus, beginning family nurse interviewers, through the use of these skills, will be able to engage a family, assess, explore, and identify strengths/problems, and make a decision to intervene or to refer the family. The nurse is also able to recognize the importance of the termination phase of therapeutic family interviewing. These stages of a family interview, with their accompanying skills, are another useful blueprint for nurses working with families.

REFERENCES

Alberta Association of Registered Nurses (AARN). (1991). *Nursing practice standards.* Edmonton, Alberta: Author.

Allred, G. H., & Kersey, F. L. (1977). The AIAE, a design for systemically analyzing marriage and family counseling: A progress report. *Journal of Marriage and Family Counseling, 2,* 131–137.

Cecchin, G. (1987). Hypothesizing, circularity, and neutrality revisited: An invitation to curiosity. *Family Process, 26*(4), 405–413.

Cleghorn, J. M., & Levin, S. (1973). Training family therapists by setting learning objectives. *American Journal of Orthopsychiatry, 43,* 439–446.

Falicov, C. J., Constantine, J. A., & Breunlin, D. C. (1981). Teaching family therapy: A program based on training objectives. *Journal of Marriage and Family Therapy, 7,* 497–505.

Figley, C. R., & Nelson, T. S. (1989). Basic family therapy skills, 1: Conceptualization and initial findings. *Journal of Marital and Family Therapy, 15*(4), 349–366.

Goren, S. (1979). A systems approach to emotional disorders of children. *Nursing Clinics of North America, 14,* 457–465.

Gurman, A. S., & Kniskern, D. P. (1981). Family therapy outcome research: Knowns and unknowns. In A. S. Gurman and D. P. Kniskern (Eds.), *Handbook of family therapy* (pp. 742–776). New York: Brunner/Mazel.

Haley, J. (1987). *Problem-solving therapy.* San Francisco: Jossey-Bass.

Hanson, S., & Heims, M. L. (1992). Family nursing curricula in U.S. schools of nursing. *Journal of Nursing Education, 31*(7), 303–308.

Janzen, S. (1980). Taxonomy for development of perceptual skills. *Journal of Nursing Education, 19,* 33–40.

Kniskern, D. P., & Gurman, A. S. (1979). Research on training in marriage and family therapy: Status, issues, and directions. *Journal of Marriage and Family Therapy, 5,* 83–94.

Liddle, H. A. (1991). Training and supervision in family therapy: A comprehensive and critical analysis. In A. S. Gurman & D. P. Kniskern (Eds.), *Handbook of family therapy* (pp. 638–697). New York: Brunner/Mazel.

Selvini-Palazzoli, M., Boscolo, L., Cecchin, G., & Prata, G. (1978). *Paradox and counterparadox.* Northvale, NJ: Jason Aronson.

Selvini-Palazzoli, M., Boscolo, L., Cecchin, G., & Prata, G. (1980). Hypothesizing, circularity and neutrality: Three guidelines for the conductor of the session. *Family Process, 19,* 3–12.

Tomm, K., & Wright, L. M. (1979). Training in family therapy: Perceptual, conceptual, and executive skills. *Family Process, 18,* 227–280.

Watson, W. L. (1992). Family therapy. In G. M. Bulechek & J. C. McCloskey (Eds.), *Nursing interventions: Essential nursing treatments* (2nd ed., pp. 379–391). Philadelphia: W. B. Saunders.

Wright, L. M. (1994). Live supervision: Developing therapeutic competence in family systems nursing. *Journal of Nursing Education.*

Wright, L. M., & Bell, J. M. (1989). A survey of family nursing education in Canadian Universities. *Canadian Journal of Nursing Research, 21,* 59–74.

Wright, L. M., Watson, W. L., & Bell, J. M. (1990). The Family Nursing Unit: A unique integration of research, education and clinical practice. In J. M. Bell, W. L. Watson, & L. M. Wright (Eds.), *The cutting edge of family nursing* (pp. 95–109). Calgary, Alberta: Family Nursing Unit Publications.

CHAPTER 6

HOW TO PREPARE FOR FAMILY INTERVIEWS

The question, "How do I prepare for family interviews?" is frequently asked by nurses who work in all types of settings. For some nurses, there are chance family meetings. For others, interviews are a planned event. For all (both the nurse and the family), the first interview is often anxiety-laden. The purpose of this chapter is to help reduce the nurse's anxiety by discussing how to plan for the first and subsequent interviews. How to develop hypotheses is addressed. Concrete issues are then presented, such as how to decide about the interview setting, who will be present, and telephone contact with the family.

HYPOTHESES

Prior to meeting the family for the first time, the nurse should develop an idea of the purpose of the interview. For example, if she is going to conduct the interview to understand how the family is coping with a chronic or life-threatening illness, it will be conducted differently than if she is trying to assess family violence or abuse or some other specified problem. In the latter example, the problem has already been identified by either the family or some other agency. Another purpose for an interview could be for the nurse to discover the family members' desires about how they would like to be involved in the patient's hospitalization. Depending on the purpose of the interview, the types of questions asked and the flow of the therapeutic conversation may be quite different.

In our clinical supervision with nurses, we have encouraged them prior to the interview to generate hypotheses related to the purpose of the meeting. Several authors have defined hypotheses. In their landmark work, Selvini, Boscolo, Cecchin, and Prata (1980) refer to a hypothesis as a formulation based on information the clinician processes regarding the family to be interviewed. They believe that a hypothesis establishes a starting point for tracking relational patterns. Fleuridas, Nelson, and

Rosenthal (1986) define hypotheses as "suppositions, hunches, maps, explanations, or alternative explanations about the family and the 'problem' in its relational context" (p. 115). For them, the purpose of a hypothesis is to connect family behaviors with meaning and to guide the interviewer's use of questions. A hypothesis provides order for the interviewing process. It introduces a systemic view of the family and generates new views of relationships, beliefs, and behaviors. Tomm (1987) considers a hypothesis to be a "conceptual posture." This is an "enduring constellation of cognitive operations that maintains a stable point of reference which supports a particular pattern of thoughts and actions and implicitly inhibits or precludes others" (p. 7). He advocates that the interviewer adopt a posture or stance of hypothesizing to deliberately focus her cognitive resources in order to generate explanations. Preferably, the hypothesis should be circular rather than linear so as to maximize the therapeutic potential. Breunlin, Schwartz, and Karrer (1990) have defined hypothesizing as "the selection of a set of ideas drawn from one or more meta frameworks which organizes and makes understandable specific feedback offered by the system" (p. 10).

The essence of all these definitions of hypothesis is similar. A hypothesis is a tentative proposition or hunch that provides a basis for further exploration. For example, we know from stress theories (McCubbin & Figley, 1984) and from our own personal and professional experiences that the time of diagnosis of an illness is generally stressful, and often symptoms temporarily become worse (Cousins, 1979). Using this as a hypothesis, the nurse can arrange a family interview to discuss the impact of the diagnosis on the family, the family's response to the illness, and the family's expectations of the nurse. In this way, the nurse can explore family patterns of adjusting to the diagnosis. She can also explore the family members' ideas of the types of relationships they would like to have with healthcare providers. The hypothesis provides general direction for the nurse interviewer in exploring this particular family's unique adjustment to a diagnosis.

HOW TO DESIGN HYPOTHESES

Hypotheses can be formulated from many bases. They can be based on information about the family gathered during hospital admission, during visiting hours, or from the other staff. The information may consist of opinions, observations of behavior or interactive patterns, and other data. Hypotheses can also be based on the nurse's previous experience and knowledge. This experience and knowledge can be about families with similar ethnic or religious backgrounds. The nurse may recall similar problems, symptoms, or situations and similar interactive patterns of previous patients and families. She may generate a hypothesis based on knowledge about family development and life cycle stages or another conceptual framework she finds most relevant. In addition to formulating hypotheses based on information about the family or previous experience and knowledge, nurses may develop hypotheses based on whatever is salient or relevant to them about the health problem/risk that is encountered at this particular time. For example, if there has been a recent tragedy in the immediate community, the nurse may find such information relevant in generating a hypothesis for this particular family at this point.

We believe it is important for nurses to state their hypothesis explicitly and consciously prior to the interview. We do not concur with those who state that hypotheses are unnecessary. Our belief is that a nurse cannot *not* hypothesize or think about a family prior to the interview. It is important for nurses to explicate their hunches so that these thoughts may be refined and made pertinent and useful to the interview process.

The following guidelines (Table 6–1) for designing hypotheses have been adapted from the work of Fleuridas et al. (1986). We encourage nurses to design hypotheses that are useful. We do not believe there is one "correct" or "right" hypothesis. Rather, the goal is to generate useful explanations for how a family is functioning. We encourage nurses to design hypotheses that are circular rather than linear. That is, a hypothesis that includes all the components of the system (e.g., the family *and* the nurse) most likely will be more circular than one that includes *either* the nurse *or* the family. The hypothesis should be related to the family's concerns. This is important because, as stated previously, a hypothesis guides the interview. For example, if the nurse develops a hypothesis that is unrelated to the family's concerns, then she will ask questions that are irrelevant to the reason why the family came to the interview. However, we encourage nurses to design a hypothesis that is different from the family's explanation or hypothesis. For example, a family may have the explanation that Puichun is a "bad daughter" who is shirking her responsibility by not caring for her elderly mother in her own home. The nurse, on the other hand, may develop an alternate hypothesis that fits the same data. The nurse's hypothesis might be that Puichun is overwhelmed by having to take care of her two preschool children while maintaining a full-time job. Thus she is stretched to the limit in trying to take responsibility for her elderly parent. Furthermore, Puichun's elderly mother may be sensitive to her stress and thus may be reluctant to live with her.

TABLE 6–1 GUIDELINES FOR DESIGNING HYPOTHESES

- Choose hypotheses that are useful.
- Generate the most helpful explanations of the family's behaviors for this particular time.
- Understand that there are no "right" or "true" explanations.
- Include all family components to make the hypothesis as systemic as possible.
- Relate the hypothesis to the family's presenting concerns so the interview can proceed along the lines most relevant to the family.
- Make the hypothesis different from the family's to introduce new information into the system and avoid being entrapped with the family in its solutions.
- Be as quick to discard unconfirmed or unhelpful hypotheses as to generate new ones.

Adapted from Fleuridas et al (1986).

Once hypotheses have been designed, the nurse can use them to guide the interview. She can ask questions of each member and note the responses to questions, thus confirming, altering, or rejecting a hypothesis. We agree with the notion put forth by Sadler and Hulgus (1989) that the "starting point for hypotheses is arbitrary and intuitive within the bounds of scientific context and therapeutic goals, but hypotheses are *validated* by evidence and either confirmed, disconfirmed or modified" (p. 265). Hypothesizing and interviewing constitute a reciprocal cycle and are interdependent. The nurse develops a hypothesis, asks questions, converses with the family about their "problem," and gathers evidence that confirms or does not confirm her hypothesis. Table 6–2 illustrates questions that invite hypothesizing about the system and the problem (Watson, 1992). As new information is generated, the nurse modifies the previous hypothesis and evolves a more useful one. The goal of the interview is to draw on the family's resources to deal with the presenting issue. More information about how to conduct family interviews is provided in Chapter 7.

Leahey and Wright (1987) have given an example illustrating how alternate hypotheses can be generated prior to the first family meeting.

> A nurse working in an extended care facility noted that the family, especially the 9- and 10-year-old children, avoided visiting their 41-year-old mother with Huntington's disease, and that the patient's symptoms worsened around visiting days. The children seemed depressed and withdrawn every time they came to the nursing unit on their monthly visits. During case conferences, the staff wondered whether there might be a connection between the family's avoidance and the patient's flailing and head banging. They generated several hypotheses to explain why the family might be avoiding the patient and why the patient's symptoms seem to exacerbate around the time of the family visits.
>
> One hypothesis pertained to the children's belief that head banging and flailing were controllable. Perhaps the children felt that their mother was not trying to control herself so she would not have to return home to care for them. This made them angry so they avoided her. An alternate hypothesis concerned the children's conflicting loyalties toward their mother and the aunt who took care of them. Perhaps they felt that if they visited too often, their aunt might think they did not appreciate her care. Thus they spaced out their visits and acted depressed and withdrawn to demonstrate both loyalty to their aunt and affection for their mother.
>
> Yet a third hypothesis involved the children's fears of developing Huntington's disease themselves. They avoided visiting and showed sadness because of their own expectations of contracting the disease. (p. 60)

Having generated several hypotheses about the family and the problem in its relational context, the nurse arranged a meeting with the family.

TABLE 6–2 QUESTIONS THAT INVITE HYPOTHESIZING ABOUT THE SYSTEM
AND THE PROBLEM

Who
Who is in the system? Who are the key players?
Who first noticed the problem?
Who is concerned about the problem?
Who is affected by the problem? (most/least)
Who is interested in keeping things the same? (most/least)
Who referred the system?
What
What is the problem at this time?
What is the meaning that the problem has for the system/for different members of the
system?
What solutions have been attempted?
What question(s) do I feel obligated to ask?
What positive function might the symptom serve in the system?
To what question could this symptom or problem be an answer?
What beliefs perpetuate the problem?
What beliefs are perpetuated by the problem?
What problems perpetuate the beliefs?
What problems are perpetuated by the beliefs?
Why
Why is the system presenting at this time?
Why this problem for this system?
Where
Where has the information about this problem come from?
Where does the system see the problem originating?
Where does the system see the problem and the system going if there is no change/if
there is change?
When
When did the problem begin?
When did the problem occur in relation to another phenomenon of the system?
When does the problem occur?
When does the problem not occur?
How
How might a change in the problem affect other parts of the system (i.e., key players,
relationships, beliefs)?
How does a change in one part of the system affect another part of the system/the
problem?
How does the symptom maintain the system?
How does the system maintain the symptom?
How will I know when my work with this system is over?
How might my work with this system constrain the system from finding their solution?

From Watson (1992), with permission.

The purpose of the interview was to clarify how the family members
wanted to be involved with the patient and how the staff could be most
helpful to them. The nurse's hypotheses were relevant to the purpose of
the interview and were not immediately explicit. She did not know if the
frequency of the family visits was a "problem" for either the children or
the patient. Rather, the problem had been identified by the staff. Thus, the

nurse chose to frame the purpose of the meeting as one in which the staff wanted to know how they could be most helpful to both the family and the patient during the patient's hospitalization.

INTERVIEW SETTINGS

A family interview can take place anywhere: in the home (in the kitchen, in the living room, or in the patient's bedroom); in the hospital (at the bedside, in the nurse's office, or in an unused treatment room); or in the community (in an interviewing room, in an office, or on the street where a homeless family "reside").

Depending on the purpose of the clinical interview, some settings are more appropriate than others. Nurses, therefore, need to consider the advantages and disadvantages of various settings. They should be flexible in choosing a setting that is appropriate for the specific purpose of the interview.

HOME SETTING

Many nurses interview families in their home setting. There are some concrete advantages to interviewing in the home. Infants, children of all ages, and very old people are able to be present more easily. Chances are increased for meeting significant but perhaps elusive family members such as boarders, adolescents, or grandparents. Firsthand observation of the physical environment is also possible. For example, sleeping arrangements and family photographs can be seen. The nurse can also experience the family's social environment. That is, rituals of eating or who answers the doorbell can be noted.

In addition to the concrete advantages to interviewing in the home, there are also other advantages. These are particularly important if the nurse is of a different social class or ethnic background than the family. Articulate middle-class parents may report in the office or school only the most exemplary family interactions. The nurse may thus have difficulty understanding how the apparent competence of the parents and the banality of the reported parent-child incidents are in such sharp contrast to the degree of behavioral upset manifested by the child. Lower-class families sometimes have difficulty bridging the gap and explaining their situation to middle-class nurses unfamiliar with their home milieu. For example, a nurse suggests that an older woman prepare her husband several small meals a day rather than one very large meal, which he is unable to consume. The nurse did not know (and the family members were too embarrassed to mention) that they shared cooking facilities with other people in their apartment building. A home interview can thus give the nurse a clearer direction for therapeutic suggestions.

Disadvantages to using the home setting for family interviews include the increased administrative and personal cost involved in traveling. There is also the increased possibility of disruptions to the interview and the increased skill that the nurse requires to flexibly structure the interview. Nurses should also be aware that a family's home is their sanctuary. If they are asked in their own home to share intense and deep emotions, then they are often left without a retreat. For example, if there is an issue of abuse, then the nurse should anticipate that the family's affective disclosure will be quite intense. Perhaps they will need more physical and psychological space to deal with the issues than their home permits. On the other hand, if the purpose of the interview is to facilitate shared grieving following the loss of a family member, then the home setting might be ideal.

Tell the family you would like to have an interview in the home so as "to get a better feel for the situation." Explain that, in your experience, there are frequently interruptions to an interview in the home (e.g., telephone calls, neighbors dropping in, or Jasmine wanting to put on the television). Ask "How should we handle this if it comes up?" In this way, you have already set the stage for work and for a specific purpose to the interview rather than for visiting. One way to handle social offerings, such as coffee or a cold drink, is to say, "Thanks, but maybe we could work first and then have coffee afterward." The work and social boundaries are thus clearly identified and the family's sense of hospitality is not offended.

OFFICE, HOSPITAL, OR OTHER WORK SETTING

The greatest advantage to using the work setting for the interview is that this is the nurse's base. Therefore, the nurse can capitalize on an opportunity and adapt the setting to the needs of the interview. There may be fewer telephone calls or visitor interruptions. Furthermore, the nurse has a greater opportunity to obtain consultation from a colleague when she is interviewing the family in the work setting.

Disadvantages to interviewing in the work setting focus around issues of context. A family can be intimidated by the professional trappings (e.g., large institution, plush furniture, and complicated equipment) and therefore display anxiety or reluctance to talk. Frank (1991), a sociology professor with cancer, described the reluctance he and his wife had about sharing information in the hospital setting because of the lack of privacy:

> One incident can stand for all the deals I made during treatment. During my chemotherapy I had to spend three-day periods as an inpatient, receiving continuous drugs. In the three weeks or so between treatments I was examined weekly in the day-care part of the cancer center. Day care is a large room filled with easy chairs where patients sit while they are given briefer intravenous chemotherapy than mine. There are also beds, closely spaced with curtains between. Everyone can see everyone else and hear most of what is being said. Hospitals, however, depend on a myth of privacy. As soon as a curtain is pulled, that space is defined as private, and the patient is expected to answer all questions, no matter how intimate. The first time we went to day

care, a young nurse interviewed Cathie (my wife) and me to assess our "psychosocial" needs. In the middle of this medical bus station she began asking some reasonable questions. Were we experiencing difficulties at work because of my illness? Were we having any problems with our families? Were we getting support from them? These questions were precisely what a caregiver should ask. The problem was *where* they were being asked.

Our response to most of these questions was to lie. Without even looking at each other, we both understood that whatever problems we were having, we were not going to talk about them there. Why? To figure out our best deal, we had to assess the kind of support we thought we could get in that setting from that nurse. Nothing she did convinced us that what she could offer was equal to what we would risk by telling her the truth. (p. 68)

Suggestions for how beginning interviewers can maximize privacy in hospital settings are given later in this chapter.

Another disadvantage of using the institution for interviewing can be the inadvertent fostering of the belief that pathology resides in the individual—for example, "Mom's the sick one. We're only coming to help Mom get over her depression." This attitude is particularly evident if the mother has been hospitalized on a psychiatric ward. This disadvantage can be handled by using the family's willingness to "help Mom." The interviewer can reframe or discuss the mother's hospitalization in a positive light. "Perhaps your mother's hospitalization has provided the family with an opportunity to all work together in a new way." (The intervention of reframing is further discussed in Chapter 4.)

How to Use the Work Setting

Some places have elaborate interviewing rooms, but most nurses have to make do with the usual clinic setting. They may, therefore, have to negotiate with coworkers for space and privacy. We recommend that you choose a private place where you will not be interrupted. For example, an unused patient room or an office is often more quiet than a four-bed room with curtains, a visitor's lounge, or a waiting area. Remove any important equipment (e.g., machines or monitors). The discussion area should ideally be sparsely furnished with movable chairs and no big desks, couches, or examining tables. This allows family members to control their own space, move closer or further away from someone, and not worry about children touching hospital equipment. A few quiet toys, such as rubber or cloth hand puppets, and paper and crayons, should be present. Books and magazines should not be available during the interview, for they give a mixed message to the family. The participants are expected to discuss issues. They should not expect to read during the interview.

Acquaint yourself with the physical layout of the room prior to the session. This probably will increase your feelings of comfort when first meeting the family.

At the beginning of the interview, if there are children, you can say to the parents, "I'd like you to handle the children in whatever way you usually do. That will give me a better idea of what you're coping with at home." If the baby starts to cry, observe who comforts the baby. If the noise level gets beyond your tolerance, notice what tolerance level the family has. Unless absolutely necessary, try to avoid giving behavioral directives during the first interview (e.g., "Watch out for that plant" or "Don't touch Dad's chest tube"). Valuable information can be lost by imposing your standards of behavior too quickly. At the same time, it is necessary to structure the interview to avoid chaos.

At the end of the session, you can assess the influence of the work setting. Ask the family if their members behaved differently than they usually do. For example, "Did the children behave better or worse today than they usually do?" "Were people more or less talkative than usual?"

WHO WILL BE PRESENT

The decision as to who will be present for the first and subsequent interviews is an important one. It is generally determined mutually by the family members and the nurse. In our early days of working with families, we thought it imperative that *all* family members be present in order to do family interviewing. However, we have changed our thinking about this. We believe that a nurse can develop hypotheses, assess, and intervene with a system regardless of who is in the interviewing room. The number of people in the room does not reflect the unit of treatment. Rather, what is more important is how the nurse conceptualizes human problems.

We have found the work of Anderson, Goolishian, and Winderman (1986) to be very helpful in thinking about human problems. The treatment system for human problems is a language system, with boundaries marked by a linguistically shared problem. These particular language systems or "problem-determined systems" may be an individual, a couple, a family, a unit group, an organization, or any combination of people that communicates around a shared, articulated problem. "In this *problem-determined systems view,* human systems defined by social constructs (e.g., families), do not cause or make problems; communicatively shared problems mark and define the system. Social-political constructions, such as family, are constructs relevant to a particular description of human experience; they are not necessary to the definition of a treatment system" (Anderson et al. 1986, p. 7).

We find the idea of "problem-determined systems" very helpful in our clinical practice. The appropriate description for the target of treatment is the problem-determined system rather then the individual, the couple, the family, or the larger system. It allows us to avoid becoming mired in the concept of "dysfunctional" family, work group, and so forth. We do not find it useful to use the term "dysfunctional family." Those people in active communication regarding a problem are the problem-determined system. We do not believe that problem-determined systems are fixed. Rather, they are fluid, always changing, and never stable. We agree with Anderson and Goolishian (1988) that as the problem definition changes, so does the membership of people involved in describing a problem. The goal of interviewing is the dissolving of the problem.

"The role of the [nurse] is simply to engage in conversation with those who are relevant to the problem resolution in such a way that there is a co-evolved new reality, a new language system, and therefore a dissipation of the problem or shared belief that a problem exists" (Anderson et al. 1986, p. 10). Through therapeutic conversation, the nurse creates a context wherein the participants in a problem-determined system no longer distinguish what they are thinking and talking about as a "problem." The nurse knows that change has occurred when the concerned membership of a problem-determined system can think and talk of their shared problems differently.

Although we believe in problem-determined systems, we also believe that nurses beginning to interview families will generally find it easiest to invite everyone living in the household to be present for the first interview. In this way, the nurse can more easily elicit information from members who most likely have a description of the problem. Haley (1987) points out that to begin family work "by interviewing one person is to begin with a handicap" (p. 10). We believe this is generally a useful notion for nurses to consider. If the problem is a marital one, then we usually try to have the husband and wife together for the first meeting. Similarly, if it is a parenting issue, then the father, mother, and child are all invited to the meeting. The more people present, the more information it is possible to gather and the more viewpoints and descriptions of the problem can be considered. Family members at the first interview might include the young children, the grandparent "who never has much to say," and the nephew "who just moved in for the weekend." Sometimes, the most significant thing that the nurse is able to accomplish in a family interview is just to bring the whole family together in one spot at one time to discuss an important issue.

Nurses frequently question whether they should include in the initial interview psychotic family members or those who are mentally or cognitively handicapped. Generally, the answer is yes. It will provide the nurse with an opportunity to assess the impact of the psychosis or mental handicap on the family. Also, it will show the nurse how the family and individual interact to deal with the presenting problem. A clinical example may help to illustrate this point. A family requested help for their 6-year-old daughter, who was "regressing, having imaginary friends, and refusing to play with peers or go to school." During the initial interview, the little girl walked over to the door and turned the doorknob. The nurse asked her not to leave the room. In response, the family members said that she wasn't leaving but rather "was letting the cat out the door." The nurse looked a bit startled because there was not a cat in the room. The nurse then asked the other children how they knew that this was what the little girl was doing. The nurse proceeded to inquire if this is how they usually responded to the child's behavior. Had the "psychotic child" not been present, the nurse would have been unaware of the siblings' contribution to the presenting problem.

FIRST CONTACT WITH THE FAMILY

The way in which the nurse makes the first contact with the family conveys an important message to the parents and the children. By inviting each person in the household to the family interview, the nurse implicitly states that each is a significant family member. Each individual has a role to play in understanding, describing, and dealing with the problem.

The rationale for bringing in the whole family can be explained in several ways. If a baby is in the intensive care nursery, the nurse might use the following explanation. "When a baby is in the intensive care nursery, we often find that family members are concerned and often anxious as well. Bringing family members in together results in more information for the whole family on how best to help the baby." Another idea would be for the nurse to say, "In the past, we kept fathers and family members out of the delivery room and out of the hospital wards. We've recognized in recent years how important it is to have family members present for special events such as the birth of a baby. Now we recognize that it is even more important for family members to be present when there is some type of illness. Family members know and care about each other. Often they have a lot to offer each other."

Sometimes, spouses will be quite agreeable to coming for an interview but they will object either to having the children present or to taking the children out of school. One way to handle the latter problem is to have interviews before school, during the lunch hour, after school, or in the evening. If this is not possible because of the nurse's work schedule, the nurse may say, "I understand your concern about the children missing school. In my experience, though, children have a tremendous amount to contribute to a family interview. They generally feel quite relieved when they see that the family is dealing with an issue about which they may have been worrying. Schools also are usually quite agreeable to children missing an hour."

HOW TO SET UP AN APPOINTMENT

Generally, the first telephone contact sets the stage for subsequent interviews. Our advice is to pay careful attention to this contact, whether you call the family to set up an appointment or a family member calls you. Napier refers to the family member on the telephone as "the family's scout" (1976, p. 4). This scout is in pioneer country and will carry important information to the other family members about the nurse and the nurse's intentions.

The purpose of the initial telephone contact with the family is to set up an appointment for an interview, explain the rationale for involving family members, and set the structure as to who will be present at the interview. Naturally, much useful information is gained over the telephone. Telephone contact is, therefore, part of the assessment process, and the nurse should treat it as such. Following is a sample first telephone contact:

Mother: Hello.

Nurse: Mrs. Lopez, this is Louise Watkins. I'm the community health nurse in your neighborhood.

Mother: Yes.

Nurse: I understand that you have a new baby. It's our practice to come out and visit all families with new babies.

Mother: Oh, I didn't know that.

Nurse: Yes, we usually do a physical examination of the baby and discuss feeding or other concerns.

Mother: Oh, that seems like a good idea. The doctor didn't tell me much about feeding.

Nurse: Sure, we can get into that during our visit. I was just calling to set up a time that would be convenient for your family and for me. I would like to see the whole family because usually when a new baby arrives, the child has a great impact, not just on the mother but on the father and other children as well.

Mother: You can say that again! My 2-year-old usually seems to like his baby sister but last night I saw him pinch her.

Nurse: Yes, those are the kind of things that we can discuss when the whole family and I get together. The meeting will probably take about an hour. I have some time available on Tuesday, at 10:00, or on Thursday, at 3:00. Which would be best for you, your husband, and the children?

Mother: Tuesday isn't good because my son is going to the doctor that day. Thursday would be better since my husband works shifts and gets off at 2:30.

Nurse: Would a 3:00 appointment give him enough time to get home, or perhaps we should make the appointment at 3:15?

Mother: Yes, 3:15 would be better.

Nurse: I look forward to seeing you and the whole family then.

Mother: Yes, me too.

Nurse: Goodbye.

Mother: 'Bye.

In the above selection, the nurse was clear, confident, goal-directed, and accommodating. The nurse set out the purpose of the interview and who she wanted present. The nurse presented the interview in a normal context by stating that this is the agency's usual practice. The nurse took charge by identifying and introducing herself without apologies and offered specific appointment times. Furthermore, the nurse also received much information that can be useful in the family assessment:

"The doctor didn't tell me much about feeding."
"I saw [the 2-year-old] pinch her."
"My son is going to the doctor. . . ."
". . . my husband works shifts. . . ."

It is not possible to provide written guidelines to cover all the various situations that nurses will encounter in trying to set up a family interview. Each family presents different challenges; therefore, each interview must be approached with flexibility. Exceptions are almost always the rule in clinical practice. Each telephone contact demands a slightly different plan of action to invite family members to an interview and/or to elicit the family's permission for a home visit. We strongly encourage CHNs especially to plan their telephone calls and appointments so as to maximize efficiency and the possibility of engagement.

RESISTANCE AND NONCOMPLIANCE

Oftentimes in our clinical supervision with nurses, we have been asked how to deal with resistant or noncompliant families. When nurses ask this, they are generally referring to families whom they perceive as oppositional or not complying with ideas and advice that could promote, maintain, or restore health. The family is designated as "noncompliant" when they do not respond to particular nursing interventions; nurses interpret this behavior as an unwillingness or a lack of readiness to change (Wright & Levac, 1992).

We do not use the terms *resistance* or *noncompliance* anymore, as we have not found them clinically useful. Resistance was initially used to describe the client's reluctance to uncover or recover from some anxiety-filled experience. The interview's job was often to uncover this material, but when this area of the client's life was touched on, the client was seen to resist the interviewer's effort. Resistance is still generally seen as "located" in the client and is often described as something the client "does." This is a linear view that implies that problems with adherence to treatment regimens reside within individuals and families, not in the interactions or relationships between individuals (Anderson & Stewart, 1982; Wright & Levac, 1992). We disagree with this view as we see the idea of resistance as a *product* of client-interviewer interaction. We believe that resistance and noncompliance are not terms describing a unilateral phenomenon but rather an interactional phenomenon.

Rather than using the terms *resistance* or *noncompliance,* we have found the multidirectional terms *cooperation* and *collaboration* to be very clinically useful. When nurses think of how they work collaboratively with families, they are less likely to impose their will on the family. They tend to open space for the family and to be more tentative and inviting of the family's point of view.

The theory behind the "death of resistance" (de Shazer, 1984) has emerged since the first edition of this book. There has been a dramatic increase in a solution-focused orientation to interviewing (Lipchik & de Shazer, 1986; de Shazer, 1991). With the emphasis on a solution focus has come an increasing emphasis on change, cooperation, and collaboration. The binocular theory of change includes the idea that the brain receives two messages: (1) The eye's view of, for example, the problem or the solution; and (2) "news of difference" between the views of the individual eyes; this relationship develops depth perception (de Shazer, 1982). As the binocular theory of change developed, the concept of cooperating emerged. "Each family . . . shows a unique way of attempting to cooperate, and the . . . interviewer's job becomes first to describe that particular manner to himself that the family shows and, then, to cooperate with the family's way and, thus, to promote change" (de Shazer, 1982, pp. 9–10). We have found the concept of a family "uniquely cooperating" to be very clinically useful. It provides far more positive direction for our work than the negative labels of resistance or noncompliance, which previously left us stymied in our clinical practice.

HOW TO INVITE A HESITANT FAMILY MEMBER

There are several possible reasons why one spouse may be hesitant to attend the family session. Each requires a different approach on the part of the nurse. Following are a few common situations that interviewers encounter.

1. "My husband would never come to a family interview. He thinks that my mother's stroke and how to handle it are my responsibility."

Ask what the wife thinks about her husband attending the interview. If she believes her mother's chronic illness is *her* responsibility and has very little to do with her husband, then she will not be interested in trying to get her husband in for a family interview. You need to work with the wife to see if she wants to alter *her* cognitive set *before* you start talking to her about her husband.

2. "My husband wouldn't want to come to a family interview. Besides, I wouldn't know how to get him there."

If the wife would like her husband to attend but does not know how to invite him, you can explore with her why she feels her husband might be hesitant. There could be several reasons:

- He may view the problem as his wife's, not his own.
- The timing of the interview might be inconvenient.

- The thought of going to a hospital might be repugnant ("seeing all those sick people").
- The husband may be afraid of being blamed for not taking a more active role in his mother-in-law's care.

You can ask the wife if she thinks any of these feelings or thoughts might be stopping her husband from becoming involved. After she has speculated on the reasons for her husband's hesitance and her own desire for him to be present, you can coach her on ways to engage him:

- She can discuss with her husband how *she needs his help* to deal with her mother's illness.
- She can find out convenient times for her husband to come to a half-hour interview.
- She can tell him exactly where the interview will be held, for example, not in the patient's room but rather in an office.
- She can discuss how *you are most hesitant* to see only parts of the family for an interview. That is, if you just saw the wife with her mother, there could be the danger that the husband would feel left out and perhaps blamed. If he were present, however, then this could not happen. He could help you to understand more fully the relationship between his wife and her mother. She can let him know that he has a unique view of the family—a view that only he can provide. Most husbands do not like to be left out of the original planning and decision-making. Once they have a fuller understanding of the purpose of a family interview, they are often quite agreeable to attend.

When the interviewer believes the husband will attend, although it may involve a little persuading, and that the interviewer needs him to be there, then the interviewer will have little problem with absent husbands. Conversely, nurses are likely to have difficulties in this area if they are timid or inconsistent in requesting the husband's presence.

Another idea for inviting an anxious or threatened family member for an interview is to suggest that the person be invited to be present as an observer, just to see what is happening. Also, the person can come whenever he is "in the mood" as a historian, an accuracy checker, or a consultant. If these suggestions are followed, it is important to ask the "observer/historian" to react at the *end* of the interview to what the family has discussed in the session. Gradually, as the family member continues to observe sessions, that member becomes more comfortable and is willing to participate *during* the interview. This may be a particularly useful way of engaging some adolescents. The idea of telling the member "not to talk" places no direct pressure on that member to participate. Silent members are often closely attuned to the process, and when a sensitive area is broached, they forget their defensive stance and join in the process. Other times, they may remain silent but hear the information.

HOW TO DEAL WITH FAMILY NONENGAGEMENT AND REFERRAL SOURCES

If you have difficulty engaging the family on the telephone, you may need to contact the referral source. That is, physicians frequently will tell a patient on discharge, "The nurse will be out to check up on you and see how you are doing." When you contact the patient, the patient may have forgotten what the physician said, or may be confused about the purpose of the visit, or simply may not be interested in being "checked up on." Sometimes in situations of suspected child abuse, the physician may contact the nurse and ask her to "drop in on the family just to see if there is any abuse happening." You may then find yourself in an awkward situation, trying to explain the purpose of your visit to a family who may be reluctant to have you come. One way to approach this is to say: "Doctor Fishkin asked me to set up a visit with your family to discuss things about raising children. Dr. Fishkin feels that most families who have infants and preschoolers as close together as yours are sometimes find it helpful to talk to the nurse." You have clearly indicated that it is on Dr. Fishkin's request that you are calling and you have attempted to normalize the purpose of the interview. If, however, the family is still reluctant to have you visit, initiate contact with the physician and have the physician set the stage for future work with the family. You should not consider this inability to engage a family as your "fault" or the family's resistance, but rather as a problem of inadequate preparation by the referral source.

Several other ideas have emerged over the past few years about dealing with referral sources. Colapinto (1988) advises interviewers to avoid focusing prematurely on family dynamics if the request for the interview comes from another agency or if the interview is compulsory. He suggests that treatment failure often ensues because of powerful conflict between the family and the referral source. We have also found this in our own clinical work. In such situations, we recommend that the nurse engage with the family and conceptualize their work together as collaboration to deal not with family issues per se but rather with dynamics between the family and the agency. In this way, the interviewer can join with the family around a problem such as "that school is always making trouble for us." Thus the focus of the nurse's work would not be on family dynamics but on work with the family to "get the school off their case." Selvini (1985) also has talked about the problem of the sibling as the referring person. She advocates that special attention be paid to the influence of this person (generally a "most competent and prestigious family member") on the nurse-family contract. Gesuelle-Hart, Kaplan, and Kikoski (1990) have recommended that the interviewer identify and grapple with the expectations of the person referring the "problem family" for assessment. They suggest some useful questions to ask:

Why is this referral being made to me at this time?
What is the relationship between the referral source and my agency?
Who is paying, for whom, for what?
What are the expectations of the hierarchy I work within?
If the referral source is unhappy with the assessment, who will hear about it?
If I am unhappy about the assessment process, who will hear about it? (p. 2)

In any situation where there is nonengagement, it is important to realize that the reluctance is important information about the dynamics between the interviewer and the family. The hypothesized reason why a person is not present should be explored at the first interview. For example, we were once asked to consult with the family members of a 59-year-old woman who was terminally ill with cancer. The hospital staff nurse arranged the interview for a time convenient for the husband and adult daughter. Only the daughter and the mother, however, showed up for the interview. In exploring the reasons why the husband did not attend, we discovered that he was 73 years old and in poor health himself, a fact unknown to the hospital staff. In asking the adult daughter about the impact of her mother's illness, we also discovered information about the father's absence. The daughter wept openly about her mother's impending death. She then stated, "If you think I'm a basket case, you should see my father. He's in worse shape than I am." Thus, in this situation, the husband's absence from the interview provided important information about the family's emotional state. It is important for nurses to understand reluctance as a systems phenomenon rather than an individual issue. We hypothesized in this case that not only was the father reluctant to attend but that the adult daughter was trying to protect him.

CONCLUSIONS

In preparing for family interviews, it is important for nurses first to remind themselves of the purpose of the meeting and then to develop hypotheses related to this purpose. Decisions about the interview setting and who will be present flow from ideas about who has a description of the problem and who is a customer for change. Table 6–3 outlines areas for nurses to consider in preparing for family interviews.

TABLE 6–3 STEPS IN PREPARING FOR FAMILY INTERVIEWS

- Design hypotheses related to purpose of interview.
- Choose appropriate interview setting.
- Decide who to invite to the interview.
- Invite family members.

REFERENCES

Anderson, H., & Goolishian, H. (1988). Human systems as linguistic systems: Preliminary and evolving ideas about the implications for clinical theory. *Family Process, 27*(4), 371–394.

Anderson, H., & Goolishian, H., & Winderman, L. (1986). Beyond family therapy. *Journal of Strategic and Systemic Therapies, 5*(4), 1–13.

Anderson, C., & Stewart, S. (1983). *Mastering resistance.* New York: Guilford Press.

Breunlin, D., Schwartz, R., & Karrer, B. (1990). The "metaframeworks" perspective in action. *Family Therapy Case Studies, 5*(2), 9–30.

Colapinto, J. (1988). Avoiding a common pitfall in compulsory school referrals. *Journal of Marital and Family Therapy, 14*(1), 89–96.

Cousins, N. (1979). *Anatomy of an illness as perceived by the patient.* New York: Bantam Books.

de Shazer, S. (1982). *Patterns of brief family therapy: An ecosystemic approach.* New York: Guilford Press.

de Shazer, S. (1984). The death of resistance. *Family Process, 23*(1), 11–16.

de Shazer, S. (1991). *Putting difference to work.* New York: W. W. Norton.

Fleuridas, C., Nelson, T., & Rosenthal, D. (1986). The evolution of circular questions: Training family therapists. *Journal of Marital and Family Therapy, 12*(2), 113–127.

Frank, A. (1991). *At the will of the body: Reflections on illness.* Boston: Houghton Mifflin.

Gesuelle-Hart, S., Kaplan, L., & Kikoski, C. (1990). Assessing the family in context. *Journal of Strategic and Systemic Therapies, 9*(3), 1–13.

Haley, J. (1987). *Problem-solving therapy.* San Francisco: Jossey-Bass.

Leahey, M., & Wright, L. M. (1987). Families and chronic illness: Assumptions, assessment and intervention. In L. M. Wright & M. Leahey (Eds.), *Families and chronic illness* (pp. 55–76). Springhouse, PA: Springhouse.

Lipchik, E., & de Shazer, S. (1986). The purposeful interview. *Journal of Strategic and Systemic Therapies, 5*(1), 88–99.

McCubbin, H., & Figley, C. (Eds.). (1984). *Stress and the family: Vol. 2. Coping with catastrophic stress.* New York: Brunner/Mazel.

Napier, A. (1976). Beginning struggles with families. *Journal of Marriage and Family Counseling, 2,* 3–12.

Sadler, J., & Hulgus, Y. (1989). Hypothesizing and evidence-gathering: The nexus of understanding. *Family Process, 28*(3), 255–268.

Selvini, M. (1985). The problem of the sibling as the referring person. *Journal of Marital and Family Therapy, 11*(1), 21–34.

Selvini, M., Boscolo L., Cecchin, G., & Prata, G. (1980). Hypothesizing—circularity—neutrality: Three guidelines for the conductor of the session. *Family Process, 19*(1), 3–12.

Tomm, K. (1987). Interventive interviewing: 1. Strategizing as a fourth guideline for the therapist. *Family Process, 26*(1), 3–14.

Watson, W. L. (1992). Family therapy. In G. M. Bulechek & J. C. McCloskey (Eds.), *Nursing interventions: Essential nursing treatments* (2nd ed., pp. 379–391). Philadelphia: W. B. Saunders.

Wright, L. M., & Levac, A. M. (1992). The non-existence of non-compliant families: The influence of Humberto Maturana. *Journal of Advanced Nursing, 17,* 913–917.

CHAPTER 7

HOW TO CONDUCT FAMILY INTERVIEWS

Once the nurse and family have decided to meet for an interview, the nurse can consider how to conduct the meeting. Just as there are stages to the whole interviewing process, there are also stages to initial interviews. An awareness of these stages provides the nurse with a general interview structure and can help to allay the nurse's anxiety.

In this chapter, we present guidelines for each stage of an initial interview. Following this, we address the stages involved in the entire interviewing process.

GUIDELINES FOR INITIAL INTERVIEWS AND ASSESSMENT

The following stages generally occur in initial interviews:

1. *Engagement stage,* in which the family is greeted and made comfortable.
2. *Assessment stage*
   a) **Problem identification** in which the nurse explores the family's presenting concerns.
   b) **Relationship between family interactions and health problem,** in which the nurse explores the family's typical responses to the health problem.
   c) **Attempted solutions,** in which the family and nurse talk with each other about solutions and their effect on the presenting issues.
   d) **Goal exploration,** in which the nurse draws together the information and the family specifies what goals, changes, or outcomes they are seeking.
3. *Termination stage,* in which the nurse and family end the interview.

ENGAGEMENT STAGE

During the engagement, or first stage of the interview, the nurse must establish a therapeutic relationship with the family. The goal in this stage is to establish an alliance between the family members and the nurse. In the beginning, the nurse is perceived as a stranger, unknown and potentially helpful or not. Because family members do not know what to expect from the nurse, she must establish herself in a relationship with the members by demonstrating understanding, competence, and caring.

We encourage nurses to consider the type of relationship that they would like to establish with families over the course of time. Thorne and Robinson (1989) have described various stages of the evolution of relationships between families experiencing chronic illness and their healthcare professionals: "naive trust," "disenchantment," and "guarded alliance." They propose that naive trust between the chronically ill, their families, and healthcare providers is inevitably shattered in the face of unmet expectations and conflicting perspectives. Anxiety, frustration, and confusion often result in disenchantment. Trust can then be reconstructed on a more guarded basis so that the chronically ill patient, the family, and the nurse can continue to engage in healthcare activities. Thorne and Robinson (1989) state that this reconstructed trust is highly selective and is based on revised expectations of the roles of both patient and provider. They suggest that there are four relationship types in guarded alliance: "hero worship," "resignation," "consumerism," and "team playing." In hero worship and team playing, the trust dimension is high, whereas in resignation and consumerism, it is low. Both team playing and consumerism highly value competence, whereas hero worship and resignation put a low value on competence.

Reciprocal trust is a very critical dimension to consider during the engagement phase of family interviewing. The nurse helps the patient and family to feel more confident in their own competence in managing illness. To develop a high degree of trust in the nurse, the patient and family are invited to explicitly state their expectations for healthcare. The nurse provides the opportunity for family members to express their desires. A high degree of trust by the patient and family in their own competence requires that their own resources be acknowledged by family members and by the healthcare providers.

When initiating engagement, the nurse should assume a position of neutrality or curiosity. Cecchin (1987) draws connections between neutrality/curiosity and hypothesizing. He maintains that curiosity is a delight in the invention and discovery of multiple patterns. "Curiosity helps us to continue looking for different descriptions and explanations, even when we cannot immediately imagine the possibility of another one . . . hypothesizing is connected to curiosity. Hypothesizing has more to do with technique. Curiosity is a stance, whereas hypothesizing is what we do to try to maintain this stance" (p. 411). We believe that curiosity nurtures circularity and is useful in the development of hypotheses. We have found hypothesizing, circularity, and curiosity to be extremely important components of our clinical work. We agree with Cecchin (1987), who states that "circular questioning can be understood as a method by which a clinician creates curiosity within the family system and therapy system" (p. 412). We have found that by using hypothesizing, circularity, and curiosity, we have become more open to families and they in turn have developed more reciprocal trust with us. The family perceives the nurse as curious when she does not take sides with any one member or subgroup. The nurse who is curious is seen as aligned with everyone and no one in particular at the same time. She is seen as nonjudgmental and accepting of everyone.

To enhance engagement, the nurse must provide structure, be active and empathic, and involve all members of the family. To provide structure, the nurse might say something such as, "We'll meet now for about 15 minutes so that I can get a better sense of your expectations and any concerns you have about hospitalization. Then I'll take a break for a few minutes to think about what you've said, after which I'll return. We can then talk about what I might be able to help you with. How does that sound to you?" By stating the structure at the beginning of the meeting, the nurse reduces the family's anxiety about how long they will meet and also gives some direction for the conversation. If possible, we recommend that a nurse take a 5-minute break after interviewing the family so that she can collect her thoughts and respond most appropriately to the family's concerns. We have adapted this idea of a break from the Milan family therapy team, who have what they refer to as an "intersession break" (Tomm, 1984).

One way in which the nurse can be active during the engagement phase of the interview is to find out who is present. Many times we have found that "extra" family members attend interviews in the hospital. On the inpatient mental health unit at Holy Cross Hospital in Calgary, we have found a compliance rate of 94 percent of families attending meetings when they have been invited (Leahey, Stout, & Myrah, 1991). These data have held constant over a 7-year period. Oftentimes, family members show up for the meeting and the nurse was not aware they were in the family. For example, extended family or ex-spouses have been invited by other family members or the patient, who believes it is important for them to be present. Another way that nurses have found useful to start an interview is to work with the family in constructing a genogram or ecomap (Chapter 3). Families generally find constructing a genogram an easy way to involve themselves in giving the nurse relevant information. At the start of the interview the nurse should ask questions of each member. We recommend that initially nurses should attempt to spend an equal amount of time with each family member. We suggest that the nurse ask the same question or a similar one to gather each person's ideas about a particular topic.

ASSESSMENT STAGE

During the assessment stage, the nurse explores four areas: problem identification, relationships between family interaction and the health problem, attempted solutions, and goals.

Problem Identification and Exploration

During this next phase of the family interview, the nurse asks the family about its main concerns, complaints, or problems. That is, what is the problem that the family is most concerned about at this time? Following the exploration of each family member's perception of the most pressing concern, we have found it useful to ask the "one question question" (Wright, 1989). That is, "If you could have only one question answered in our work together, what would that one question be?" This is a particularly effective way to elicit the family's deepest concerns at the beginning of the clinical work. It provides a focus for the conversation and generates new information between family members and between the nurse and the family. For example, the husband of a 44-year-old woman newly diagnosed with multiple myelomas asked, "How can I support my wife and children better during this time?" The teenage daughter asked, "How can I learn more about my mother's illness?" The patient asked, "'How long do I have to live?" The young adult son asked, "Should I avoid having my friends come over to the house so as to keep it more quiet for my mother when she returns home?" It is evident from the four questions asked by the family members that they each had a different expectation for the interview and for their relationship with the nurse.

Fleuridas, Nelson, and Rosenthal (1986) recommend that the family's definition of the concern be elicited by focusing on the three time frames of past, present, and future. Within each time frame, the nurse can ask questions pertaining to areas of difference, areas of agreement and disagreement, and explanations as to the meaning of the concern. It is important to emphasize that an effective interview does not depend on the use of any one type of question but rather on the knowledge of when, how, and to what purpose questions are used with particular family members at particular points in time.

Leahey and Wright (1987) have given the following examples of how to elicit the family's concerns by asking circular questions focusing on the present, past, and future.

Present. The nurse should ask each family member, including the children, to share their knowledge and understanding of the present situation. For example, the community health nurse working with a diabetic family could ask such questions as:

- What is the family's main concern *now* about John's diabetes?
- How is this concern a problem for the family *now* as compared to before?

- Who agrees with you that this is a problem?
- What is your explanation for this?

Past. In exploring the past, the nurse can again ask questions pertaining to:

- *Differences:* (How was John's behavior before his diabetes was diagnosed?)
- *Agreement/disagreement:* (Who agrees with Dad that this was the main concern when the family lived in Seattle?)
- *Explanation/meaning:* (What do you think was the significance of John's decision to stop injecting his own insulin?)

Future. During the initial interview with a new family, the nurse must learn about the family' own hypotheses or beliefs about the problems (Tomm, 1984). In asking the family to explain the present situation, the nurse should consciously attempt to identify previously unrecognized connections. This might be done by asking such questions as:

- If Bill suddenly developed renal disease, how would things be different from the way they are now?
- Does Bill agree with you?
- If this were to happen, how would you explain the change in John's relationship with Mom? (pp. 62–63)

If the nurse finds that children or adolescents are reluctant to identify concerns in the family, she may need to ask the children alternate questions. Children may hesitate to disagree with their parents' description of the situation. A nurse can ask a child what he or she would like to see different in the family or how he or she would know if the problems went away. For example, one 8-year-old repeatedly stated that there were no difficulties surrounding his brother's diabetes and his mother's overinvolvement with the sick child. However, when the nurse asked a future-oriented question about what differences he would notice in the family if his brother did not have diabetes, the 8-year-old said that he and his mother could go to basketball games after school. At the time of the interview, the mother had stated she was hesitant to leave the house after the boys returned from school for fear that her oldest son would have an insulin reaction.

Other ideas for involving children in interviews have also been presented. Benson, Schindler-Zimmerman, and Martin (1991) suggested modifications of circular questions to be used with young children. These modifications based on Piagetian theory take into account the cognitive developmental limitations of children. For example, they suggest that relationship differences can be explored by providing props such as scarves, hats, and glasses for the children. The role-play technique using

TABLE 7–1 FACTORS TO CONSIDER IN DEFINING THE PROBLEM

1. Presenting Problem
   - Specify
2. Problem Identification
   - Who in the family was the first to identify the problem? And then who?
   - When was problem identified?
   - Concurrent life events/stressors at time of identification of problem
   - Who else (family members, friends) agrees that it is a problem? Who disagrees?
   - How does the family understand that this problem developed (beliefs)?
3. Problem Evolution
   - What behaviors became problematic?
   - Pattern of development
   - Frequency of problem emergence
   - Time intervals of quiescence
   - Factors aggravating
   - Factors alleviating
   - Who in the family is most/least concerned?

Adapted from Family Nursing Unit records, Faculty of Nursing, University of Calgary.

props enables children and adults to display their perceptions. Another idea would be to give the child an ordered array of pictures ranging from a frowning face to a smiling face. The nurse could then ask, "Which one of these is most like how you and your brothers got along this week?" (p. 367).

In exploring the presenting concern, the nurse should obtain a clear and specific definition of the situation. Table 7–1 lists some factors for the nurse to consider when defining the problem. The nurse can identify conflict among family members about the problem definition if this arises. When differences exist, then the nurse clarifies the issues further to help define the problem for which the family is seeking change.

The nurse can also ask questions of each member about his or her own explanation for the situation *now.* For example, what is their explanation or hypothesis about why this problem exists at this point in time? Furman and Ahola (1988) have given a number of useful suggestions for exploring the family's causal explanations for its own and other people's behavior. They suggest that the simplest way to do this is to ask direct, explanation-seeking questions such as, "What do you think is the reason for your son's psychosis?" Another idea is to ask the clients to use their imagination to discuss an explanation. The interviewer can also offer a variety of alternative explanations or "gossip in the presence" by asking triadic questions such as, "What do you, Donald, think is Pat's explanation for your mother's depression?" In exploring the family's preexisting explanations, it is essential that the interviewer be curious and avoid agreeing or disagreeing with the explanation. Furman and Ahola (1988) suggest that there are several advantages to exploring the family's causal explanations, including improving cooperation between the interviewer and the family, developing systemic empathy with all family members versus selective empathy with one or two, detaching oneself from explanations provided by other professionals, recognizing and avoiding coalitions, loosening firmly held explanations, diluting negative explanations, and attaining an ability to speculate with the clients about the effects of believing in one explanation or the other.

Relationship between Family Interaction and the Health Problem

Once the main problems have been identified, the nurse asks questions about the relationship of family interaction to the health problem. Table 7–2 lists some factors to consider in exploring family interaction related to the presenting problem. The nurse conceptualizes the information she has already gathered from the family in light of the hypotheses generated prior to the interview and begins to develop additional questions. These questions focus on *interactional* behaviors dealing with the three time frames of present, past, and future. Within each time frame, the nurse once again explores differences, agreements/disagreements, and explanations/meanings. It is important to emphasize that the purpose of asking these questions is not merely to gather data. Rather, the nurse and the family are coauthoring a new story to replace a problem-saturated description (White & Epston, 1990). That is, by asking circular questions, the nurse generates new ideas and explanations for herself *and* for the family to consider.

Present. In exploring the present situation, the nurse could ask: "Who does what, when? Then what happens? Who is the first to notice that something has been done?" The nurse steers away from asking about traits supposedly intrinsic to a person, for example, being "shy." Rather, the nurse might ask, "When does he *act* shy?" or "Who does he *show* shyness to?" Then, "What does Ashley do when Carley shows shyness?"

The nurse can inquire about differences between individuals: "Who is better at getting grandmother to make her meals, Shanghi or Puichun?" The nurse can also inquire about differences between relationships: "Do your ex-husband and Danielle fight more or less than your ex-husband and Nadiya?" In working with families with chronic or life-threatening illness, the nurse should explore differences before or after important events or

---

TABLE 7–2 FACTORS TO CONSIDER IN EXPLORING FAMILY INTERACTION RELATED TO THE PROBLEM

- Current manifestations of the problem.
- Typical responses of family members and others to the problem.
- Other current associated problems/concerns.
- How does the problem influence family functioning?
- How do family members understand that they have not been successful in conquering this problem (beliefs)?

Adapted from Family Nursing Unit records, Faculty of Nursing, University of Calgary.

milestones. For example, the nurse could inquire: "Do you worry more, less, or the same about your wife's health since her emergency surgery?"

In addition to exploring areas of difference, the nurse can inquire about areas of agreement/disagreement: "Who agrees with you that Brandon is the most forgetful in giving your mother eye drops three times a day? Who disagrees with you?" The nurse should explore the family's explanation for the sequence of interaction: "How do you understand Brandon's tendency to be most forgetful about the eye drops? Are there ever times that he does remember? What seems to be different about the times he remembers?"

Past. In exploring the past, the nurse uses similar types of questions to explore:

> Differences: How was it different? How does that differ from now?"
> Agreement/disagreement: "Who agrees with Len that Dad was more involved in Lori Ann's exercise program?"
> Explanation/meaning: "What does it mean to you that after all this time, things between your wife and her mother have not changed?"

In addition to exploring how the family saw the problem in the past, we have found it extremely useful to explore how they have seen changes in the problem. Weiner-Davis, de Shazer, and Gingerich (1987) have found that change in the problem situation frequently occurs prior to the first meeting with the interviewer. Families can often recall and describe such changes, if prompted. It is important to note that often the family must be prompted to emerge from their problem-saturated view of the situation. For example, a man may tell the nurse at the community mental health center that his male partner drinks very heavily and has always done this "until recently." If the nurse is attuned to inquiring about pretreatment changes, then she will ask questions about the differences that the man has noticed recently. For example, she might inquire, "Is his recent behavior the kind of change you would like to continue to have happen?" The idea of noticing exceptions to problems is one that we have used frequently in our clinical work, and we are indebted to de Shazer (1982, 1991) and White (1990) for emphasizing it.

Future. By focusing on the future and how the family would like things to be, the nurse instills hope for more adaptive interaction regarding the presenting concern. She also co-constructs a reality between family members and herself for a "problem-dissolved system" (Anderson & Goolishian, 1988). The nurse can ask questions pertaining to:

> Differences: "How would it be different if your grandfather didn't side with your mother against your father in managing Luke's Crohn's disease?"
> Agreement/disagreement: "Do you think your mother would agree that if your grandfather stayed out of the discussions, things would be better?"

Explanation/meaning: "Dad, if your wife stopped phoning her father for advice about Luke's Crohn's disease, what would that mean to you?"

During this part of the interview, the nurse attempts to gain a systemic view of the situation and a description of the full cycle of repeated interactions. These interactions may be between family members or between family members and the nurse. We stress that it is not important for the nurse to understand or agree with the problem but rather to be curious. She should be able to describe the sequence of the development of the problem over time and the current contextual problem interaction, as well as the times when the problem does not show itself.

Attempted Solutions

During this next phase of the assessment, the nurse explores the family's attempted solutions to the problem. Table 7–3 lists some factors to consider when exploring the family's attempted solutions. The process can begin with general questions related to the problem. For example, "How have you tried to obtain information from physicians and nurses about Emma's condition in previous hospitalizations?" More specific questions should then be used to identify the least and most effective solutions for achieving what the family desires. The nurse can ask when these solutions were employed. For example, "What was least helpful in trying to get information from the nurses? What was most effective?" The nurse can ask if any successful elements in the solutions are still being employed, and, if not, why not. Similar types of sequences of interaction questions that focus on difference, agreement/disagreement, and explanation/meaning can be used to explore the family's attempted solutions to the presenting concerns.

White (1991) has discussed the idea of attempted solutions as "unique outcomes." These are experiences that contradict the client's dominant or problem-saturated story. Unique outcomes provide a window to what might be considered to be the alternative territories of a person's life. "For an event to comprise a unique outcome, it must be qualified as such by the persons to whose life the event relates" (p. 30). It must be

---

TABLE 7–3 FACTORS TO CONSIDER IN EXPLORING THE FAMILY'S ATTEMPTED SOLUTION

- How has the family tried to resolve the problem?
- Who tried?
- With whom?
- What results?
- What were the events precipitating the search for professional help?
- Who is most in favor of agency help? Most opposed?
- What was the sequence of events resulting in actual contact with the agency?

Adapted from Family Nursing Unit records, Faculty of Nursing, University of Calgary.

judged to be important and significant and represent a preferred outcome and an appealing development that people are attracted to as a new possibility. He recommends "re-authoring," in which the interviewer can ask a variety of questions to facilitate the process of preferring unique outcomes. For example, White (1991) suggests the following questions:

- How did you get yourself ready to take this step?
- What preparations led up to it?
- Just prior to taking this step, did you nearly turn back?
- If so, how did you stop yourself from doing so?
- Looking back from this vantage point, what did you notice yourself doing that might have contributed to this achievement?
- What developments have occurred in other areas of your life that may relate to this?
- How do you think these developments prepare the way for you to take these steps? (p. 30)

White also discusses the value of what he calls "experience of experience questions." Such questions "invite persons to reach back into their stock of lived experience and to express certain aspects that have been forgotten or neglected with the passage of time" (p. 32). They "recruit the imagination of persons in ways that are constitutive of alternative experiences of themselves" (p. 32). Examples include:

"If I had been a spectator to your life when you were a younger person, what do you think I might have witnessed you doing then that might help me to understand how you were able to achieve what you have recently achieved?"

"What do you think this tells me about what you have wanted for your life, and about what you have been trying for in your life?"

"How do you think that knowing this has affected my view of you as a person?"

"Exactly what actions would you be committing yourself to if you were to more fully embrace this knowledge of who you are?"

"If you were to side more strongly with this other view of who you are, and of what your life has been about, what difference would this make to your life on a day to.day basis?" (p. 32)

In working with families dealing with life-threatening or chronic illness, the nurse should be aware of additional "helping agencies" involved in healthcare delivery. We have found it important to ask such questions as, "Have any other agencies attempted to help you with this problem? What has been the most useful advice that you have received? Did you follow this advice? What has been the least helpful advice?" Leahey and Slive (1983) point out the usefulness of exploring the differing ideas espoused by the helping systems. If there is unclear leadership or a confused hierarchy within the helping systems, the family can be placed in a conflictual situation that is similar to that of a child whose parents continually disagree. Confusion among helping agencies can exacerbate the family's concerns. In this way, the attempted solution (assistance by helping agencies) can become an entirely new problem for both the family and other agencies. It is important for the nurse to be aware of whether this situation exists before she attempts to intervene.

Goal Exploration

At some point during the interview, the nurse must establish what goals or outcomes the family expects as a result of change. Table 7–4 lists some factors for nurses to consider when exploring goals. We believe that families are seeking practical results when they come to a healthcare provider; families are pragmatists. They are "in pain" or "suffering" and their desire is to get rid of a problem. The problem may be between themselves as family members or the problem may be between the family and the nurse (e.g., the family desires practical information about the acceptable level of physical activity following a myocardial infarction [MI] and the nurse has not provided such concrete information). Family members may expect a large change (e.g., "My brother Sheldon will be able to walk without the aid of a cane") or a small but significant change, such as, "We will be able to leave our handicapped daughter with a babysitter for 1 hour a week."

In many cases, a small change is sufficient. We believe that a small change in a person's behavior can have profound and far-reaching effects on the behavior of all persons involved. Experienced nurses are aware that small changes lead to further progress. de Shazer (1991) indicates that workable goals tend to have the following general characteristics. They are:

(1) small rather than large
(2) salient to clients
(3) described in specific, concrete behavioral terms
(4) achievable within the practical contexts of clients' lives
(5) perceived by the clients as involving their "hard work"
(6) described as the "start of something" and not as the "end of something"
(7) treated as involving new behavior(s) rather than the absence or cessation of existing behavior(s). (p. 112)

Goals describe what will be present or what will be happening when

TABLE 7–4 FACTORS TO CONSIDER WHEN EXPLORING GOALS

- What general changes does the family believe would improve the problem?
- What specific changes?
- What are the expectations of how the agency may facilitate change in the problem?

Adapted from Family Nursing Unit records, Faculty of Nursing, University of Calgary.

the complaint or concern is absent. We believe that unidimensional behavioral goal statements, such as "I will be eating less," are not as desirable as multidimensional, interactional, and situational goal statements that describe the "who, what, when, where, and how" of the solution. Such a multidimensional goal statement might be, "I will be eating a small, balanced meal in the evening at the dinner table with my husband and we will not be watching television but rather talking to each other."

There are many ways in which the nurse can clarify the family's goals with such future/hypothetical questions as, "What would your parents do differently if they did not stay at home every evening with Frazer?" The nurse can explore future/hypothetical areas of difference ("How would your parents' relationship be different if your dad allowed your uncle to take care of Frazer one evening a week?"), areas of agreement/disagreement ("Do you think your Dad would agree that your parents would probably have little to talk about if they went out one evening a week?"), and explanation/meaning ("Tell me more about why you believe your parents would have a lot to talk about when they went out that one evening a week. What would that mean to you?").

Hewson (1991) has elaborated an interesting idea of combining past and future questions. She terms these "past prediction questions." For example, "if you were to tell me next week (month/year) that you had done X, what could I find in your past history that would have allowed me to predict that you would have done X?" (p. 10). "The questions capitalize on the 'possibility to probability' phenomena at the same time as inviting a richer account of the past history of the new/old story" (p. 10).

We have found it particularly useful in our clinical work to ask the "miracle question" (de Shazer, 1988) to elicit the family's goals. de Shazer (1991) describes the question in this way:

> Suppose that one night there is a miracle and while you are sleeping the problem . . . is solved: How would you know? What would be different?
> What will you notice different the next morning that will tell you there has been a miracle? What will your spouse notice? (p. 113)

The miracle question elicits interactional information. The person is asked to imagine someone else's ideas as well as their own. The framework of the miracle question (and others of this type) allows family members to bypass their causal explanations. They do not have to imagine how they will get rid of the problem, but rather can focus on results. de Shazer (1991) states that "this then allows them to bring more of their previous non-problem experiences into the conversation; thus, the goals developed from the miracle question are not limited to just getting rid of the ~~problem/complaint~~.* Clients frequently are able to construct answers to this 'miracle

---

*To emphasize the elimination of the problem, de Shazer often strikes out the word problem or complaint.

question' quite concretely and specifically. 'Easy, I'll be able to say 'no' to cocaine.' 'She'll see me smile more and go to work with more enthusiasm'' (p. 113).

Nurses working with families with a member with a chronic or life-threatening illness often find family members quite vague about the changes they expect. For example, "We would like Jordan to feel good about himself even though he has had a colostomy." Experienced clinical nurses know that "feeling good about oneself" is very difficult to describe or measure. We recommend that the nurse should ask the family to describe the smallest concrete change that Jordan could make to show that he "feels good about himself." By asking for this degree of specificity about desired change early in the nurse-family relationship, we believe it is more likely that the family and nurse can accomplish the desired change.

TERMINATION STAGE

There are several ways in which the nurse knows when to close the initial interview or assessment. Most likely, she and the family will have engaged and begun to develop a working relationship. She will have completed the assessment stage. The nurse and the family have collaboratively delineated their concerns. Family interaction related to the concerns has been explored. Attempted solutions and their results on the presenting problems have been elicited. Goals, changes, and outcomes for both the family and the nurse have been delineated.

GUIDELINES FOR THE REMAINING INTERVIEWING PROCESS

Once the nurse has completed the initial interviews or assessment, she can consider the entire interviewing process. The stages of the interviewing process generally include:

1. Engagement
2. Assessment
3. Intervention
4. Termination

Having discussed assessment and presented guidelines for conducting initial interviews, we will now address the remaining stages of the interviewing process. We will present guidelines for planning, intervening, and terminating with families.

PLANNING

After an initial assessment is completed, a beginning nurse interviewer frequently worries about whether or not to intervene with a family. The following questions often arise: Am I the appropriate person to offer intervention? Do I have sufficient skills? Or perhaps, should another professional, such as a social worker, psychologist, or family therapist, be called in?

Does every family that is assessed need further intervention? This is not to say that interventions only begin at the intervention stage. Rather, they are part of the total interview process from engagement to closure. For example, just by asking the family to come together for an interview, the nurse has intervened. Each time the nurse asks a circular question, she influences the family, generates new information, and intervenes.

For nurses, the decision to offer additional intervention, refer the family to others, or discharge them is a complex one. Several factors need to be examined before making the choice: the level of the family's functioning, the level of the nurse's competence, and the work context.

Level of the Family's Functioning

The nurse should recognize the complexity of the case. Christophersen (1979) advocates that treatment begin if the referring problem has been detected early and clearly defined procedures for management have been published. Most nurses would agree with this position but would find it very idealistic. Community health nurses and mental health nurses, in particular, often work with families who are not referred early. Some of these families who present have an unusual number of physical and emotional problems and frequently are involved in one crisis after another. These families offer specific challenges to the clinician.

Our recommendation is that nurses should carefully assess the family's level of functioning and its desire to work on specific issues, such as management of hemiplegia following a stroke, impact of cystic fibrosis on the family, negotiation of services for the elderly, or caring for a special-needs child. If the family is at all amenable to working on such an issue, then it is incumbent on the nurse to either offer intervention or help them to get appropriate assistance by referring them to others. Guidelines for the referral process are given in Chapter 9.

Grace and Camilleri (1981) discuss the ethical issues involved in who should be treated. They point out that "with the popularizing of psychiatry, a surface inspection would seem to indicate that everyone is in need of psychotherapy in one form or another" (p. 565). The childless couple, the family with young infants, the family with adolescents, the single-parent family, and the aging family are all considered to be candidates for psychotherapeutic aid. Many people lead psychologically constricted and difficult lives but should they be "treated"? This is a troublesome question for helping professionals.

Our recommendation is that nurses must ethically weigh two opposing positions when they make the decision to intervene with, refer, or discharge a family. One position states that if a person is potentially dangerous to self or others, then that person should receive intervention. On an individual level, a suicidal patient is such an example. On a larger system level, a child-abusing family is an example. An opposing position has been voiced by Szasz (1973). He asserts that the individual should decide for himself or herself whether to be treated or hospitalized. A person's self-responsibility is vehemently defended. Szasz's position on individual rights can be extrapolated to cover a family's rights. Today, many families that previously were considered deviant are seen to be functioning adaptively, such as sole-parent adoptive families or homosexual couples. It is our hope that nurses will ethically and wisely consider the family's level of functioning. This is a necessary step prior to deciding whether or not to offer further treatment. In Chapter 9, we present some ideas that we have used when we have decided not to offer additional treatment to families.

Level of the Nurse's Competence

The nurse should consider her personal and professional capacity when choosing to work with a family. If the nurse has experienced a recent death of a family member, the nurse may not be able to facilitate appropriate grieving in family members. Likewise, if the nurse has strong views that people with psychosomatic illnesses are hypochondriacs, then the nurse would be best advised not to attempt work with such families. We do not subscribe to the view that a nurse has to have personally dealt with a situation (e.g., raised teenagers) to be of help to a family. Most noteworthy in a nurse is clinical competence. We do believe, however, that the nurse should attempt to be well informed and not just offer advice that might or might not be helpful. On a professional level, the nurse needs to evaluate her competence. Am I at the beginning or the advanced level of family interviewing skill? Can I obtain supervision to aid in dealing with complex families? Each nurse should examine these questions and the answers prior to making a decision about intervening with families.

Work Context

Sometimes considerable controversy is raised about the issue of who is competent to treat clients (Koeske, Koeske, & Mallinger, 1993). This controversy involves issues of definition and professionalism. How a "family problem" and how a "medical problem" are defined in a particular work setting can fuel the controversy. If a nurse (working with a patient who had a stroke) invites the relatives to come for a class, is the nurse treating a family or treating a medical problem? We take the approach that the definition of the problem is less important than the solution. That is, if the whole family is involved, then the definition of the problem is a question of semantics.

The issue of professional territoriality is a very thorny one with no pat answers. Sometimes the patient sees the psychologist for psychodiagnostic testing and the social worker to deal with the family and outside agencies. The role of the nurse with the family in this situation can become controversial. If the nurse does a family assessment and decides to intervene with the family, is the nurse usurping the social worker's position? Or perhaps, is the nurse usurping the physician's position by making the decision to intervene? Another development that we view as too constricting is the use of the term "medical family therapy" (McDaniel, Hepworth & Doherty, 1992). This type of language, particularly the use of the word "medical," can inadvertently exclude or diminish nursing's involvement with families (Bell, Wright, & Watson, 1992). There are no simple answers to complex professional and territorial issues. We urge nurses to work cooperatively to ensure the best family care possible. In general, we believe the best person to intervene in a situation is the one with the most ready access to the system level in which the problems manifest themselves. However, we believe that in the past, nurses have been too quick to turn over family care to other professionals. Nurses are now reclaiming their important role in providing family-centered care.

INTERVENTION STAGE

Once the nurse has decided to intervene with the family, we recommend that she review CFIM (Chapter 4). This will stimulate her ideas about change, and she can then design interventions to trigger the particular domain of family functioning affected: cognitive, affective, or behavioral.

In choosing interventions, we encourage nurses to attend to several factors to enhance the likelihood that the interventions will trigger change in the desired domain of family functioning. These factors are outlined in Table 7–5. First, the intervention should be related to the problem the nurse and the family have contracted to change. Second, the intervention should be derived from the nurse's hypothesis about the problem and domains of family functioning. Third, the intervention should match the family's style of relating. (We have found in our own clinical work that sometimes we are biased toward one particular domain of family functioning, such as cognitive or affective, and that we have thus erred in devising interventions that we are most comfortable with rather than ones that the family may find most useful.) Fourth, the interventions should be linked to the family's strengths. We believe that families have inherent resources and that the nurse's responsibility is to invite families to use these resources in new ways to tackle the problem. Fifth, the interventions should be consistent with the family's ethnic and religious beliefs. Sixth, the nurse should devise a few interventions so that she can consider their relative merits. For example, are

---

TABLE 7–5 FACTORS TO CONSIDER WHEN DEVISING INTERVENTIONS

- What is the agreed-on problem to change?
- What domain of family functioning is the intervention aimed at?
- How does the intervention match the family's style of relating?
- How is the intervention linked to the family's strengths and previous useful solution strategies?
- How is the intervention consistent with the family's ethnic and religious beliefs?
- How is the intervention new or different for the family?

---

they new ideas for the family or are they "more of the same" solutions the family has already tried? We do not believe that there is one "right" intervention. Rather, there are only "useful" or "effective" interventions. In our experience, we have found that a nurse sometimes reaches an impasse, with a family not changing, when the nurse persists *either* in using the same intervention over and over *or* in switching interventions too rapidly.

Once the nurse has devised an intervention, she must attend to the executive skills (Chapter 5) required to deliver the intervention. Part of the success of any intervention is the manner in which the intervention is given. The family requires confidence that the intervention will promote change. The nurse also needs to show that the *nurse has* confidence and belief that the intervention or task requested will benefit the family.

However, interventions need to be tailored to each family; therefore, the preamble or preface to the actual intervention will vary. For example, if a family is feeling very hopeless and frustrated with a particular problem, the nurse might want to say, "I know this might seem like a hard thing that I'm going to ask you to do, but I know your family is capable. . . ." On the other hand, if the nurse is making a request of a family who tends to be quite formal with one another, then the nurse might preface it with, "What I'm going to ask you to do may make you feel a little foolish or silly at first, but you'll notice as you do it a few times that you will become more comfortable."

When giving a particular assignment to a family between sessions, it is a good idea to try and include all family members. Haley (1987) suggests that one way to make this possible is to think of the assignment as you would any other piece of work. Therefore, it requires some family members needed to do the "job," someone to supervise, someone to plan, and another family member to check if the job gets done.

Sometimes, it is necessary to review with the family members what the particular assignment is in order to check their understanding of what is being requested. Reviewing the assignment is a good idea, whether it is something to be carried out within the interview or between interviews. If assignments or experiments are given to be completed between sessions, then the nurse should always ask for a report at the next interview. If the family has not completed or only partially completed the assignment, then the reason needs to be explored.

We do not subscribe to the view that families are noncompliant or resistant if they do not follow our requests. Rather, we become curious about their decision to choose an alternate course and try to learn from their response. We believe family interviewing is a circular process. The nurse intervenes, and the family responds in its unique way. The nurse then responds to this response and the process continues.

During the intervention stage, the nurse must be aware of the element of time. How useful or effective an intervention is can only be evaluated after the intervention has been implemented. With some interventions, change may be noted immediately. However, it is more common that changes will not be noticed for a lengthy period of time. Just as most problems occur over time, problems also need an appropriate length of time to be resolved. It is impossible to state how long one should wait to ascertain if a particular intervention has been effective, but changes within family systems need to filter through the various system levels.

More information about devising interventions is provided in Chapters 4 and 8.

TERMINATION STAGE

The last stage of the interviewing process is known as termination or closure. It is critically important for the nurse to conceptualize how to end treatment with the family so as to enhance the likelihood that changes will be maintained. In Chapter 5, we outlined the conceptual, perceptual, and executive skills useful for the termination stage. In Chapter 9 we address in depth the process of termination and focus on how to evaluate outcome.

CLINICAL CASE EXAMPLE

Following is an example of how a nurse conducted family interviews using the guidelines we have given in Chapters 6 and 7.

PREINTERVIEW

Developing Hypotheses

The Home Health Agency received a referral on the Auerswald family for home nursing services, physiotherapy, nutrition counseling, and mental health counseling. Mr. Auerswald, 51, was a paraplegic and in a wheelchair because of multiple traumas suffered in an industrial accident. He was unemployed. Mrs. Auerswald, 49, a homemaker, was the primary caretaker. She was reported to be depressed. The home-care nurse hypothesized that Mrs. Auerswald's depression could be related to feeling overresponsible for caring for her husband. The nurse wondered what the husband's role might be in perpetuating this. She was also curious to know what other social and professional support systems were involved and what their beliefs were about the family's health problems. During the course of the family interview, the nurse found much evidence from both the husband and wife to confirm the usefulness of her initial hypothesis. She used this hypothesis to provide a framework for her conversation with the couple.

Relation to CFAM. The nurse generated her hypothesis based on knowledge of and clinical experience with other families in similar situations and with a similar ethnic background. It was also based on the structural category of CFAM (internal and external family structure, ethnicity), the developmental category (middle-aged families), and the functional category (roles, circular communication, beliefs).

Arranging the Interview

The wife stated that she did not want to discuss her depression with the nurse while her husband was awake. The nurse requested that for the first home visit that husband and wife be interviewed together. The couple agreed to this.

Relation to CFAM. The nurse elaborated her thinking about family roles and speculated that Mrs. Auerswald may be protecting her husband from her problem. In terms of the CFAM category of verbal communication, the nurse speculated that there might not be clear and direct communication between the husband and wife.

INTERVIEW

Engagement

The genogram data revealed that:

- The husband and wife are alone in the city; extended families and children live in other cities and visit infrequently.
- The wife had been married previously and had stayed with her first husband for 18 years although he physically abused her. She thought it was her responsibility to protect her children.
- This was husband's first marriage.

Relation to CFAM. The above information added some support for the nurse's initial hypothesis in terms of the wife's beliefs about responsibility and an isolated family structure.

Assessment

Problem Definition. Mrs. Auerswald described the problem as "my husband has had such a hard tragedy, but now I'm the one who is depressed. It doesn't make sense." Mr. Auerswald described the problem as his wife's "worrying too much."

Relationship between Family Interaction and Health Problem. By asking circular questions, the nurse elicited that the wife had not allowed herself a break in caretaking for 2 years. The husband encouraged her to "go out and meet people," but she stated that she was fearful he might be too lonely if she met other people. Mr. Auerswald stated that this would not be a problem for him. They both reported that recently Mrs. Auerswald had become depressed. She cried frequently and had difficulty sleeping.

Mrs. Auerswald takes excellent physical care of her husband and bathes him daily. He is appreciative of all her nursing care. She feels guilty to ask for help from his parents.

Attempted Solutions. Mrs. Auerswald had recently visited her family doctor, who prescribed antidepressant medication for her. She had requested home-care services once before, but she said that because "their schedule is unreliable [and she] never know[s] when they are coming," she had discontinued treatment with the nurses. On the advice of her physician, Mrs. Auerswald agreed to try Home Care again.

Relation to CFAM. The nurse noted that the Auerswald's problem-solving approaches were directed toward either self-sufficiency or professional resources outside the family. They sought help from the family doctor and from the home-care agency only infrequently, and they were reluctant to call on extended family for assistance.

Goals. Mrs. Auerswald's desire was to "not feel depressed, [to] feel good about myself." The smallest significant change that she was able to describe was to be able to "go out one afternoon a week without feeling guilty." Mr. Auerswald was in agreement with his wife's goals.

Intervention

Consideration of CFIM. Having developed a useful, workable hypothesis that fit the data from the family assessment, the nurse began to consider interventions with Mr. and Mrs. Auerswald in the cognitive, affective, and behavioral domains of family functioning. The focus of intervention was Mrs. Auerswald's depression.

Interventions and Outcome. Knowing that Mrs. Auerswald had stayed in a physically abusive first marriage for 18 years in order to protect her children, the nurse asked questions about beliefs and feelings of overresponsibility. The nurse triggered change in Mrs. Auerswald's beliefs by asking both husband and wife behavioral effect, triadic, and hypothetical questions about responsibility. She asked the couple to engage in behavioral experiments to try out new ways of being self-responsible. Both Mr. and Mrs. Auerswald challenged their own beliefs about depression being a solely biological problem and began to take more responsibility for their own lives. Mr. Auerswald stated he only wanted a bath three times a week. Mrs. Auerswald requested caretaking help from her mother-in-law and was able to leave her husband alone for 2 hours, three times a week while she played cards with friends. The couple reported significant improvement in her depression. The home-care agency continued to provide nursing and physical therapy services for the family. The nurse and home health aide focused on supporting the couple's new beliefs about appropriate responsibility.

CONCLUSIONS

Guidelines for nurses to consider during initial interviews and also during the whole process of interviewing have been delineated. We recommend that nurses use these guidelines as ideas and suggestions for how to maximize the effectiveness of their time with families. We caution nurses, however, to remember the uniqueness of every family situation and we encourage them to use guidelines with sensitivity to each clinical situation.

REFERENCES

Anderson, H., & Goolishian, H. (1988). Human systems as linguistic systems: Preliminary and evolving ideas about the implications for clinical theory. *Family Process, 27*(4), 371–394.

Bell, J. M., Wright, L. M., & Watson, W. L. (1992). The medical map is not the territory; or, "Medical Family Therapy?"—Watch your language? *Family Systems Medicine, 10*(1), 35–39.

Benson, M., Schindler-Zimmerman, T., & Martin, D. (1991). Assessing children's perceptions of their family: Circular questioning revisited. *Journal of Marital and Family Therapy, 17*(4), 363–372.

Cecchin, G. (1987). Hypothesizing, circularity, and neutrality revisited: An invitation to curiosity. *Family Process, 26*(4), 405–414.

Christophersen, E. (1979). Behavioral pediatrics. In D. Hymovich & M. Barnard (Eds.), *Family health care* (Vol. 1, pp. 354–372). New York: McGraw-Hill.

de Shazer, S. (1982). *Patterns of brief family therapy: An ecosystemic approach.* New York: Guilford Press.

de Shazer, S. (1988). *Clues: Investigating solutions in brief therapy.* New York: W. W. Norton.

de Shazer, S. (1991). *Putting difference to work.* New York: W. W. Norton.

Fleuridas, C., Nelson, T., & Rosenthal, D. (1986). The evolution of circular questions: Training family therapists. *Journal of Marital and Family Therapy, 12*(2), 113–127.

Furman, B., & Ahola, T. (1988). The return of the question "why": Advantages of exploring pre-existing explanations. *Family Process, 27*(4), 395–410.

Grace, H., & Camilleri, D. (1981). *Mental health nursing: A socio-psychological approach* (2nd ed.). Dubuque, IA: W. C. Brown.

Haley, J. (1987). *Problem-solving therapy* (2nd ed.). San Francisco: Jossey-Bass.

Hewson, D. (1991). From laboratory to therapy room: Prediction questions for reconstructing the "new-old" story. *Dulwich Centre Newsletter, 3*, 5–12.

Koeske, G. F., Koeske, R. D., & Mallinger, J. (1993). Perceptions of professional competence: Cross-disciplinary ratings of psychologists, social workers and psychiatrists. *American Journal of Orthopsychiatry, 63*(1), 45–54.

Leahey, M., & Slive, A. (1983). Treating families with adolescents: An ecological approach. *Canadian Journal of Community Mental Health, 2*(2), 21–28.

Leahey, M., Stout, L., & Myrah, I. (1991). Family systems nursing: How do you practice it in an active community hospital? *Canadian Nurse, 87*(2), 31–33.

Leahey, M., & Wright, L. M. (1987). Families and chronic illness: Assumptions, assessment and intervention. In L. M. Wright & M. Leahey (Eds.), *Families and chronic illness* (pp. 55–76). Springhouse, PA: Springhouse.

McDaniel, S. H., Hepworth, J., & Doherty, W. J. (1992). *Medical family therapy.* New York: Basic Books.

Szasz, T. (1973). *The myth of mental illness.* New York: Harper & Row.

Thorne, S. E., & Robinson, C. A. (1989). Guarded alliance: Health care relationships in chronic illness. *Image, 21*(3), 153–157.

Tomm, K. (1984). One perspective on the Milan systemic approach: 2. Description of session format, interviewing style and interventions. *Journal of Marital and Family Therapy, 10*(3), 253–272.

Weiner-Davis, M., de Shazer, S., & Gingerich, W. J. (1987). Building on pretreatment change to construct the therapeutic solution: An exploratory study. *Journal of Marital and Family Therapy, 13*(4), 359–364.

White, M. (1991). Deconstruction and therapy. *Dulwich Centre Newsletter, 3*, 21–40.

White, M., & Epston, D. (1990). *Narrative means to therapeutic ends.* New York: W. W. Norton.

Wright, L. M. (1989). When clients ask questions: Enriching the therapeutic conversation. *Family Therapy Networker, 13*(6), 15–16.

CHAPTER 8

HOW TO DOCUMENT FAMILY INTERVIEWS

It is important for the nurse to devise a system for integrating and recording the large amount of complex data gathered in the family interviews. Such a system provides the nurse with an organized and clear overview of the family. Using this overview, the nurse can then decide which are key issues to focus on and which issues are tangential. With an organized recording system, the nurse is able to move back and forth from macroscopic to microscopic data, and the family receives more holistic healthcare. The purpose of this chapter is to discuss how to integrate and record data from the nursing of families. The nurse's impressions of a family interview is addressed first. How to examine the data and use both the Calgary Family Assessment Model (CFAM) and the Calgary Family Intervention Model (CFIM) are discussed. A strengths/problems list, an initial assessment summary, and an intervention plan are also detailed. The use of progress notes for integrating and recording hypotheses, interventions, and family responses is addressed. How to record a discharge synopsis is presented. The issue of confidentiality of records also is discussed.

INITIAL IMPRESSIONS

There are many factors that affect the nurse's first response to an initial family interview. External factors might include how cold or warm the interview room is, how dirty or clean it is, how noisy the surrounding area is, and so forth. Internal factors have an even more profound influence on the nurse's evaluation. Inherent within each nurse are her self-image, value system, mores, prejudices, attitudes, and past personal and work life experiences, as well as her unique way of perceiving other individuals. These internal factors strongly influence the nurse's response to a family.

The nurse's response must be recognized as important data. Too often in the past, nurses have strived for a purely clinical response to an individual or a family. They were either embarrassed, ashamed, or most likely did not recognize how their personal thoughts and feelings influenced their clinical judgment. We recommend that a nurse consciously take a few minutes following an interview to blurt out (even if only to herself) personal initial reactions to a family interview. These quick "gut reactions" can then be dealt with as the nurse formally starts to integrate the data. In our experience, interviewers who are able to quickly "discharge" their personal reactions about a family have a far easier time integrating the data. The *unacknowledged* initial hypotheses or responses are the most mischievous.

The following case scenario illustrates a nurse's initial reactions to a family interview. The family is composed of husband, Leroy, age 28, who is a roofer; wife, Melvina, age 27, who works part-time in a dry cleaners; and children, Junior, age 3½, and Vicki, age 9 months. The couple has been married for 6 years. When Junior was examined in the outpatient clinic, his speech was found to be approximately 8 months delayed and it was noted that he was small for his age. The nurse also noticed the difficulty that the mother had in controlling Junior when he was running up and down the halls. After the clinic session, the interdisciplinary team made the following plans: the physician would continue with the physical investigations, the nurse would arrange for a family interview to discuss Junior's difficulties, and the team would reconvene for a conference in 2 weeks.

Mr. and Mrs. Hamilton, Junior, and Vicki attended the initial interview. Immediately following the interview, the nurse said:

> So much crying! I would have been so frustrated with Vicki. I could never have been so nice to her as Mrs. Hamilton was! Mr. Hamilton never once offered to take the baby or help out.
> The poor parents, they've got so many problems with their extended family. No wonder they feel "maybe we're doing something wrong as parents."
> They're awfully critical of Junior—never had a good word to say about him.
> Junior's darling, friendly too. Gave me a hug on the way out.
> They jump around a lot in their conversation. I'm not sure what really is the issue, Junior's misbehavior or his lack of eating. They never mentioned his delayed speech.

In voicing these quick reactions, the nurse was able to express her own anxiety and feelings of empathy, compassion, and frustration. She was also reminded of her own family and how her ex-husband did little to support her when their infant was crying. The nurse was aware, therefore, that she had to safeguard against a tendency to feel overly sympathetic toward the wife and overly critical toward the husband.

In summary, we recommend that nurses acknowledge their feelings and immediate reactions to family members. Having done so, they can then decide to either discard the feelings or use them appropriately. For example, the nurse *used* her own initial impressions of the Hamiltons in the following way:

> The baby's prolonged crying may stimulate frustration in the father and Junior. I'll explore this in the future.
>
> Given the relationship with their extended family, the parents are probably exquisitely sensitive to being blamed. I must watch my tone of voice and choice of words so that I don't inadvertently blame them.
>
> Junior's hugs may indicate that he's hungry for attention. It would be inappropriate for him to receive much attention from me because I'm not available to him consistently. Also, the parents may feel I'm usurping their position if I give him lots of praise. I'll try to encourage the parents to do this.
>
> The parents are quite concerned but seem to be under a lot of stress. Maybe that's why the conversation jumped around a lot. I'll try to keep the next interview more focused.

Having acknowledged her initial impressions, the nurse can proceed to review the content *and* process of the interview by using CFAM. The content of the interview refers to the concrete communication, the "what" that is stated. The process refers to the "how," implying movement. Process is a dynamic concept, whereas content is static. The process is not the activity *per se,* but the way in which the activity is carried out. An example of *content* from the Hamilton interview is the description of the grandparents' interfering with the couple's management of the children. The *process* of the discussion was that Mrs. Hamilton became sad and tearful while her husband tried to minimize the problem: "Ah, she gets too emotional with the folks all the time. The best thing is to forget about what they say and live your own life."

RECORDING SYSTEM

There are many different kinds of tools a nurse can use to record family interviews. Some are fairly specific, whereas others are more general. The ideal recording tool should above all be consistent with the nurse's interviewing practice. That is, if the thrust of the family interview is to obtain information about medication compliance, then considerable space should be allocated for this data. Second, the record should provide an integrated picture of family strengths and problems. Too much emphasis on problems or constraints can lead to overinvolvement and intrusion by the nurse. It can also foster dependency by the family. Third, an assessment record should be a springboard for developing an intervention plan. Isolated bits of information, such as "the mother is experiencing depression," or "the father is unemployed," need to be drawn together into a composite picture. Strengths need to be linked to the problem so they can be used as resources for problem-solving. From this integrated picture, a plan of action emerges. Without this picture, the deficiencies and gaps in the data are obscured. Lastly, the recording system should be able to be easily used by the nurse interviewer. Most nurses have heavy workloads and become frustrated if they have to fill out lengthy forms.

The recording system that we recommend is fairly general. It can be adapted to almost any agency's or hospital's philosophy and any style of nursing practice. The system consists of six parts:

1. CFAM
2. Strengths/problems list
3. Family assessment summary
4. CFIM
5. Progress notes
6. Discharge summary

Before dealing with each part separately, we would like to strongly emphasize the conceptual skills that are involved in integrating the data following an interview. Nurses must think in a critical fashion to integrate data; that is, they must sort through all the information and generate ideas about its meaning. They must distinguish between observation and inference. They must be willing to entertain hypotheses and equally be willing to discard them as new data emerge that are inconsistent with their first hypothesis. In deciding which information to include and which to discard, nurses engage in the processes of deliberation, judgment, and discrimination. The task of integrating and recording the data is not an easy one. It requires intellectual discipline.

How to Use the Calgary Family Assessment Model

As we discussed in Chapter 3, CFAM is an integrated conceptual framework consisting of three major categories: structural, developmental, and functional. Each category contains several subcategories. It is useful to conceptualize the three assessment categories and the many subcategories as a branching diagram (Fig. 8–1). As the nurse uses the subcategories on the right of the branching diagram, she collects more and more microscopic data. It is important for the nurse to be able to move back and forth on the diagram to draw together all relevant information into an integrated assessment. For example, the nurse may explore boundary issues in depth with a family. The nurse thus obtains microscopic data within the structural category of the assessment model, and she needs to be able to integrate this with other data within the diagram. Isolated microscopic statements such as "The parental subsystem has a diffuse boundary" have little meaning and are of limited help in devising an intervention plan. In combination with other data, however, this statement may become particularly rich and meaningful: "The parental subsystem has had a diffuse boundary since Nydia was born with Down syndrome and the grandmother began to care for her." In this example, structural, developmental, and functional data are combined:

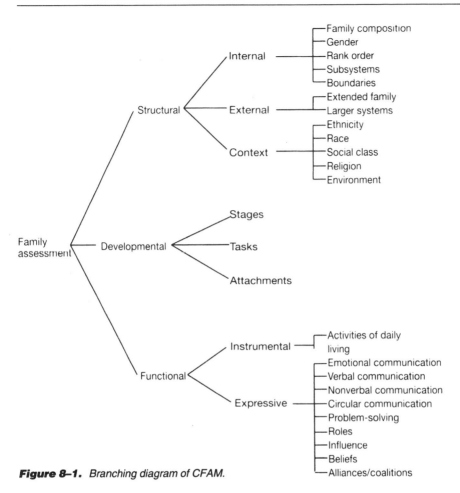

Figure 8–1. Branching diagram of CFAM.

Structural: parental subsystem diffuse boundary
Developmental: stage of families with young children
Functional: grandmother assumes parenting role

Following an initial interview, it is important for the nurse to mentally review each category. In this way, the nurse gains a macroscopic view of the family.

After reviewing the family structure outline (the top branch of Fig. 8–1) the nurse should examine the family genogram and ecomap. It will help the nurse to conceptualize *this particular family* and how it differs from or is similar to other families. The Hamilton family, for example, is a young, nuclear, working-class family with the mother working part-time while the father works full-time. The family boundary seems fairly permeable, with much interface with the extended families of origin. Subsystem boundaries are clear.

TABLE 8–1 THE DEVELOPMENTAL CATEGORY OF CFAM: SAMPLE FAMILY
LIFE CYCLE VARIATIONS

- Middle-class North American
- Divorce and postdivorce
- Remarried and stepfamily
- Professional and low-income
- Adoptive
- Other types

In addition to an understanding of the family structure, who is in it and how they fit into their context, the nurse requires an understanding of how *this* family came to be at *this* stage in its developmental life cycle (Table 8–1). We recommend that the nurse review the stages and tasks appropriate to the family's specific developmental life cycle (e.g., Table 8–2; see also Tables 3–2 through 3–4). Also, we suggest that the nurse draw a diagram illustrating family attachments. The Hamilton family attachment diagram is given later in this chapter.

While reviewing the developmental category, the nurse can identify the normative as well as the crisis issues that the family dealt with during each stage. For example, the Hamilton family is currently in Stage 3 (Families with Young Children). They have adjusted the marital system to make space for children. During Stage 2, they had to deal with the unexpected death of Mrs. Hamilton's brother. This influenced their marital relationship by creating emotional distance between the couple. Also, the relationships with their families of origin were not adequately defined during Stage 2. These past difficulties in Stage 2 are having repercussions for task achievement in Stage 3. Hence, they are of current significance.

When the nurse has mentally examined the CFAM structural and developmental categories, she can then review the family functioning category. This third CFAM category is detailed in Table 8–3.

For the Hamilton family, the nurse can identify strengths as well as difficulties in the area of expressive functioning, particularly emotional and circular communication; influence; and coalitions.

The nurse need not be too microscopic in the review of CFAM categories. If the nurse uses too many subcategories, she may become overwhelmed by the complexity of the data. It is important for the nurse to maintain a macroscopic, integrated, metaview of the family. After the nurse has used the CFAM several times, the categories will be familiar.

How to Develop a Strengths/Problems List

Having reviewed CFAM, the nurse should identify family strengths and problems in the structural, developmental, and functional categories. Using the interview data base, the nurse should then prepare a strengths/problems list and indicate issues at whatever system level the nurse presently conceptualizes them. Thus, the nurse will have completed three steps in integrating the assessment data: (1) review CFAM, (2) identify

TABLE 8–2 MIDDLE-CLASS NORTH AMERICAN FAMILY LIFE CYCLE STAGES AND TASKS

Family Life Cycle Stage	Emotional Process of Transition: Key Principles	Second-Order Changes in Family Status Required to Proceed Developmentally
1. Leaving home: Single young adults	Accepting emotional and financial responsibility for self	1. Differentiation of self in relation to family of origin 2. Development of intimate peer relationships 3. Establishment of self re: work and financial independence
2. The joining of families through marriage: The new couple	Commitment to new system	1. Formation of marital system 2. Realignment of relationships with extended families and friends to include spouse
3. Families with young children	Accepting new members into system	1. Adjusting marital system to make space for child(ren) 2. Joining in childrearing, financial, and household tasks 3. Realignment of relationships with extended family to include parenting and grandparenting roles
4. Families with adolescents	Increasing flexibility of family boundaries to include children's independence and grandparents' frailties	1. Shifting of parent-child relationships to permit adolescent to move in and out of system 2. Refocus on midlife marital and career issues 3. Beginning shift toward joint caring for older generation
5. Launching children and moving on	Accepting a multitude of exits from and entries into the family system	1. Renegotiation of marital system as a dyad 2. Development of adult-to-adult relationships between grown children and their parents 3. Realignment of relationships to include in-laws and grandchildren 4. Dealing with disabilities and death of parents (grandparents)
6. Families in later life	Accepting the shifting of generational roles	1. Maintaining own and/or couple functioning and interests in face of physiological decline; exploration of new familial and social role options 2. Support for a more central role of middle generation 3. Making room in the system for the wisdom and experience of the elderly, supporting the older generation without overfunctioning for them 4. Dealing with loss of spouse, siblings, and other peers and preparation for own death. Life review and integration.

From Carter and McGoldrick (1988), with permission.

TABLE 8–3 FUNCTIONAL CATEGORY OF THE CFAM

Family Functioning

A. Instrumental
   1. Activities of daily living
B. Expressive
   1. Emotional communication
     a. Types of emotions
     b. Range of emotions
   2. Verbal communication
     a. Direct versus displaced
     b. Clear versus masked
   3. Nonverbal communication
     a. Types
     b. Sequencing
   4. Circular communication
   5. Problem-solving
     a. Identification patterns
     b. Instrumental versus emotional problems
     c. Solution patterns
     d. Evaluation process
   6. Roles
     a. Role flexibility
     b. Formal versus informal
   7. Influence
     a. Instrumental
     b. Psychological
     c. Corporal
   8. Beliefs
     a. Family expectations/goals
     b. Family beliefs about problems
     c. Family beliefs about change
   9. Alliances/coalitions
     a. Directionality, balance, and intensity
     b. Triangles

strengths/problems, and (3) list strengths/problems according to system level.

There are various systems levels indicated on the strength/problems list. Community–whole-family system refers to the relationship between the family and its neighborhood or community. A problem at this system level might be, for example, that the family members are isolated and scapegoated by the community because of their race. The professional–whole-family system level depicts the relationship between the family and healthcare providers in particular but also with other professionals such as teachers or clergy. A strength at this system level might be, for example, that the family and the home-care service have developed a cooperative working relationship. The next system level is that of the nurse and the whole family. This level depicts the nature of the relationship between the nurse and the family. The relationship could be one of naive trust, disenchantment, guarded alliance (Thorne & Robinson, 1989), or some other type. The whole-family system level refers to interactions among all family members. The marital subsystem designates issues pertaining to the couple as marital partners or as parents. The parent-child system level refers to issues between the children and parents. The sibling subsystem depicts the relationship issues among brothers and sisters. The individual systems level refers to the biological, psychological, and social issues pertaining to individual family members.

Family strengths are very important to note. They can be used effectively to enhance family life. More specifically, they can be linked to problems and used as effective resources in problem-solving. Otto (1963) had identified 12 family strengths:

1. The ability to provide for the physical, emotional, and spiritual needs of the family members.
2. The ability to be sensitive to the needs of the family members.
3. The ability to communicate thoughts and feelings effectively.
4. The ability to provide support, security, and encouragement.
5. The ability to initiate and maintain growth-producing relationships and experiences within and without the family.
6. The capacity to maintain and create constructive and responsible community relationships.
7. The ability to grow with and through children.
8. The ability to perform family roles flexibly.
9. The ability for self-help and to accept help when appropriate.
10. The capacity for mutual respect for the individuality of family members.
11. The ability to use a crisis experience as a means of growth.
12. The concern for family unity, loyalty, and interfamily cooperation.

In developing a strengths/problems list, the nurse should acknowledge major structural, developmental, and functional issues that are presently affecting *family* interaction. The nurse should not try to make a perfect list but rather strive to identify the major issues. Problems frequently overlap several systems levels. It is often difficult, therefore, to differentiate whole-family problems from marital issues from individual difficulties. Under which system level a problem is placed is quite arbitrary. It does have significance, however, in that it guides which interventions are chosen. For example, a nurse could identify Mrs. Hamilton's sadness as an individual problem and list it as depression. Most likely, the intervention for this problem would then be medication or individual therapy. However, if the problem of sadness is identified as "difficulty with emotional communication" and is listed as a marital issue, then the intervention would be different. It would probably involve marital intervention to help both partners meet their needs.

We strongly recommend that beginning nurse interviewers *first* attempt to identify as many *family* strengths and problems as possible. This is, they should initially restrain themselves from listing issues under the individual category level. We find that this helps nurses to "think family." Nurses are often very accustomed to thinking of individual issues, such as the father's alcoholism or the mother's anxiety. They need to reconceptualize these problems at a higher system level if they are to deal with the *family.* Some questions that we recommend nurses ask themselves to assist in this conceptualization include:

Who is most affected by . . . (e.g., the father's drinking)?
How does that person attempt to influence the father?
Who supports that person in attempting to influence the father?
Who does not support that person's attempts to influence the father?

By thinking through these questions, the nurse will start to conceptualize the father's individual issue as a whole-family system or marital system problem.

Although we strongly recommend family assessment and intervention, we do not subscribe to the view that *all* issues are family-centered, however. Major physical, psychological, and social issues that are primarily personal in origin are listed under the individual category level. For example, Junior Hamilton's delayed speech and short stature are listed as individual problems. Mrs. Hamilton's sadness, on the other hand, is conceptualized as a marital issue, "difficulty with emotional communication." It is, therefore, listed under the marital system level. Her interest and concern about being a good parent is also listed under the marital/parental system level and not under the individual level.

Figure 8–2 shows a sample strengths/problems list for the Hamilton family.

When the nurse has identified the strengths and problems of the family, she can then begin to analyze the relationship of the family's strengths to its problems. For example, in the Hamilton family's strengths/problems list, the unresolved conflict between the couple and the grandparents is identified. Thus, the nurse should think about the following questions, "What is the relationship between the strengths and the problems?" "Is there a way that the strength can be used to deal with the problem?"

With the Hamiltons, the nurse hypothesized that the grandparents were genuinely concerned about Junior and the family but that they demonstrated their concern in a way that exacerbated the problem rather than helped it. The grandparents tended to interfere by offering advice, and the couple had not found ways to deal with this.

In evaluating the strengths/problems list, the nurse decided to leave the apparent conflictual data on the list. She reasoned that this would help

Family name: Hamilton   Date

Subsystems	Strengths	Problems
Community— whole family system	• Grandparents a possible support	• Unresolved conflict with both families of origin • Isolated—five moves in 3 years
Professionals— whole family system	• Engaged with pediatric clinic	• Reluctant to ask for information concerning Junior's health problems
Nurse— whole family system	• Guarded alliance	
Whole family system	• Strong beliefs: "We're survivors," "special family"	
Marital/parental subsystem	• Care about each other • Concerned about being good parents	• Difficulty with emotional communication—Melvina sad, shows helplessness. Leroy disconfirms.
Parent-child subsystem	• Able to bond with Vicki • Father can be positive with Junior	• Difficulty with behavior controls • Unrealistic expectations of a 3 1/2-year-old with new sibling • Isolation of Junior
Sibling subsystem	• At clinic Junior can be positive with Vicki	• Intense rivalry reported
Individual systems		• Junior—speech delay of 8 months, small stature

Figure 8–2. *Strengths/problems list: The Hamilton family.*

her to maintain a neutral stance vis-à-vis the grandparents. Furthermore, it would help her to keep a metaperspective on the Hamilton family situation. Should the nurse and the couple decide in the future to invite the grandparents in for a joint family interview, she would be aware of the boundary issue between the generations.

Having considered the relationship between family strengths and problems, the nurse should then attempt to prioritize the concerns. In most instances, the nurse and the family will have already done this during the interview. We recommend, however, that the nurse do this again after completing the strengths/problems list. In our experience with beginning family interviewers, we have found that they often become overly enthusiastic and "change oriented" when they are integrating and recording the data. Not every family needs intervention. Nor do all problems require resolution. We therefore strongly urge nurses to concentrate on the *presenting* issue. With the Hamilton family, the parents' priority concern was their difficulty with controlling Junior's behavior.

HOW TO SUMMARIZE THE FAMILY ASSESSMENT

Although the strength/problems list is a useful working tool, it does not provide a sufficient summary of the family assessment. It would probably be too cryptic and fragmented for the rest of the nursing and healthcare team to use in delivering service to a family. Table 8–4 outlines a family assessment summary. Table 8–5 presents a sample family assessment summary of the Hamilton family.

It is in the family assessment summary that the nurse must synthesize theory and practice. All the isolated questions and answers discussed in the interview are woven into a synthetic pattern. For example, the nurse hypothesized that the Hamilton couple had a symmetrical relationship when they were both able to share emotionally with Mrs. Hamilton's brother. Since his death, they have had difficulty with emotional communication. They are attempting now to have a complementary relationship with each other, whereby Mrs. Hamilton cries and expresses her feelings to her husband. It is her expectation that he in turn should provide her with support. He attempts to do this by joking around with her. However, this does not help to alleviate her sadness. Thus, they are experiencing tension in their relationship. The nurse identified this pattern and discussed it as a problem under the marital system level in the family assessment summary.

HOW TO DEVELOP AN INTERVENTION PLAN

When the nurse has reviewed CFAM, identified and listed the family's strengths and problems, and prepared an assessment, she should then develop an intervention plan. We have found the following three steps helpful when we develop intervention plans in our clinical practice:

1. Identify specific problems
2. Review the CFIM
3. Choose interventions

Each of these steps is discussed separately.

TABLE 8–4 OUTLINE OF A FAMILY ASSESSMENT SUMMARY

Family Name: _____   Date: _____
Family Members Present at Interview: _____
Interviewer: _____
Place of Interview: _____

I. Referral Route and Presenting Problem
   1 or 2 sentences summarizing reason for referral and referral source.

II. Family Composition
   Draw a genogram. Include name, age, and occupation or school grade of each member of the family. Circle those currently living at home.

III. Family Attachment
   Draw an attachment diagram. Indicate the strength and nature of the bonding among family members.

IV. Pertinent History (very brief and relevant to presenting problem)
   a. Chronological sequence of events leading to current presenting problem. Include previous solutions to cope with the problem and professional help sought.
   b. Developmental history of the family including pertinent information re: families of origin and significant personal, social, vocational, and medical events.

V. Strengths/Problems
   Identify family strengths. List family problems (structural, developmental, and functional) and individual problems (physical, psychological, and social) at their appropriate system levels.

VI. Hypothesis/Summary
   Summarize the connections between the initial hypothesis, presenting problems, pertinent history, and family strengths. If necessary, refine the hypothesis to provide direction for intervention.

VII. Goals and Plans
   Indicate plans for intervention, referral, or discharge. Indicate family's reaction and the outcome.

VIII. Signature

TABLE 8–5 FAMILY ASSESSMENT SUMMARY: THE HAMILTON FAMILY

Family Name: Hamilton_____   Date: 1/4_____

Family Members Present at Interview: Whole Family_____

Interviewer: Anne Marie Levac, RN, BS_____

Place of Interview: Children's Hospital_____

I. Referral Route and Presenting Problem
    Junior Hamilton, age 3½, and his mother were identified at the Pediatric
    Outpatient Clinic by myself and Dr. Carpenter as needing a family assessment.
    The mother had difficulty controlling his behavior (running up and down the halls)
    and appeared extremely upset.

II. Family Composition
    The family is composed of husband, Leroy, 28, a roofer; wife, Melvina, 27, who
    works part-time in a dry cleaners; and children, Junior, 3½, and Vicki, 9 months.

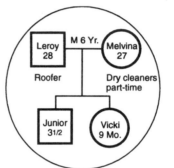

III. Family Attachment

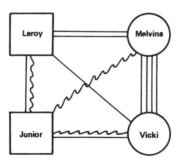

IV. Pertinent History
    Junior: Normal pregnancy and delivery and milestones to age 34 months. Speech
    delay of 8 months and small stature. Complete history on Dr. Carpenter's report.
    Family: When Junior was approximately 1 year old, parents began to have
    difficulty controlling his behavior, that is, spreading feces, refusing to listen, and
    being a picky eater. Tried toilet training him at 13 months and have tried punishing
    him by sending to his room, getting him to help clean up the mess, and spanking.
    Have also visited two other pediatric clinics for the same complaints. Report these
    visits were "not helpful."
      The couple has been married for 6 years, no separations, five moves within the
    past 3 years (two between cities). Mother's brother died when Junior was 1 year old.
    Both families of origin are heavily involved in giving conflicting advice.

Continued

TABLE 8–5 FAMILY ASSESSMENT SUMMARY: THE HAMILTON FAMILY
(Continued)

V. Strengths/Problems
  a. Community–Whole Family System
    1. Strengths
    Extended family interested. The grandparents might be available as a source of support.
    2. Problems
      (a). Unresolved conflict with both families of origin. The paternal grandparents live outside of the city but see the family about once a month. They telephone frequently and, according to both parents, imply that the children are not being raised properly. Melvina in particular feels angry at them for interfering. The maternal grandparents live in the city and, although they do not interfere as much with regard to the children, seem to imply that Melvina is not a competent mother. She apparently was overprotected as a child and feels resentful that her parents now seem to favor her sister-in-law. The couple has not found helpful ways of dealing with their anger toward their parents.
      (b). Isolation. The family has moved five times in 3 years and has no close neighbors or friends.
  b. Professionals–Whole Family System
    1. Strengths
    The family engaged readily with Pediatric Clinic. The father took time off work without pay to attend.
    2. Problems
    The parents lack information about Junior's health problems.
  c. Nurse–Whole Family System
    1. Strengths
    The parents asked about my qualifications and areas of expertise. They responded fairly quickly to a collaborative approach. We developed a guarded alliance given their feelings of mistrust with previous nurses.
  d. Whole Family System
    1. Strengths
    Family believes they are "special." They have overcome adversity in the past (e.g., unemployment, automobile accident) and are proud of being "survivors."
  e. Marital/Parental System
    1. Strengths
    Concerned re: good parenting. The couple cares a tremendous amount for each other and are concerned about being good parents.
    2. Problems
    Difficulty with emotional communication. Since the mother's brother's death, the couple has had difficulty communicating emotionally. Mrs. H. reports that her brother was "the only person we could talk to." She is sad, feels inadequate as a mother, and tends to share this by crying or expressing her helplessness. How this affects her husband is not clearly known at this time. He responds to his wife by overprotecting her, not confirming what she says, or trying to talk her out of it. This perpetuates her feelings of inadequacy. The couple report not having a satisfactory emotional relationship.

Continued

TABLE 8–5 FAMILY ASSESSMENT SUMMARY: THE HAMILTON FAMILY
(Continued)

f. Parent-Child System
  1. Strengths
     Ability to bond. The couple has been able to bond adequately with Vicki. The father can be positive with Junior and seems interested in him. The father is very concrete but seems willing to learn.
  2. Problems
     Difficulty with behavioral controls. Junior seems confused about behavioral limits and tends to act up. When he does test, his father responds by becoming frustrated and ignoring him or withdrawing. His mother feels overwhelmed, and both parents focus on the negative rather than on the positive. They have limited knowledge of normal growth and development.
g. Sibling Subsystem
  1. Strengths
     Sharing. Junior can be positive with Vicki as was evidenced with he gave her an appropriate toy during the family interview.
  2. Problems
     Intense rivalry. Junior has placed feces in Vicki's crib, bites her, pushes her, and so forth. During the family interview, no negative behavior was noticed.
h. Individual System
  1. Strengths
     Peer interaction. Junior has been attending nursery school for 3 months and according to his mother is reported to be doing well although his speech is delayed.
  2. Problems
     Health. Junior has a speech delay of 8 months. He is below the third percentile in height.

VI. Hypothesis/Summary
    Junior Hamilton, 3½, and his parents present with difficulty controlling his behavior. The problem has existed for 2½ years. One hypothesis is that the parents, unaware of normal child development, use age-inappropriate techniques. It is also hypothesized that a precipitating factor was the unexpected death of Mrs. Hamilton's brother, a close confidant of both Mr. and Mrs. Hamilton. Although the couple stated that they tried to separate their own feelings and not to displace them onto the children, it is my hypothesis that when Mrs. H. is feeling sad, she handles this by getting angry with Junior. Mr. H. "gets after" Junior particularly when he sees his wife upset. Vicki seems to stimulate and receive positive feelings from the parents while Junior encourages and receives negative feelings. The children seem triangulated into the marriage.

VII. Goals and Plans
    a. The parents and Junior agreed to meet for four sessions to learn how to manage Junior's behavior.
    b. Joint meeting with parents, Dr. Carpenter, and myself set for January 19 to discuss Junior's health, that is, short stature, delayed speech, and normal growth and development.

VIII. Signature: <u>Anne Marie Levac, RN, BS</u>

Identify Specific Problems

The intervention plan that the nurse creates will depend on the severity and complexity of the family's problems and the richness of their strengths. A problem list that indicates mild problems may reflect a family coping with a normal developmental crisis or a transient situation. If the problem list, however, suggests severe family issues, then it is essential that the nurse recognize the gravity of the situation and not offer placebos or unrealistic interim solutions for conditions that require more expert assistance. In these situations, the nurse may wish to refer the family for more specialized assistance. Suggestion for how to refer are given in Chapters 5 and 9.

If the nurse is going to continue work with the family, however, she should identify specific target problems along with the family. Priorities need to be set. It is generally unwise for the clinician to move too quickly to work on marital issues unless the couple has specifically asked for help in this area. A rule of thumb is to start with the presenting issue and try to exert the most leverage in the system; that is, the nurse should promote change where the maximum benefit will be realized by all family members. With the Hamiltons, the nurse chose to work on helping them control Junior's behavior because that was an area that concerned both parents. Also, it would enable the nurse to bring the couple together to discuss their feelings and beliefs about childrearing. In this way, the nurse would be indirectly fostering emotional communication between the spouses. In addition, she planned to have sessions with the father, the mother, and Junior to foster positive feedback. The nurse reasoned that if they had to travel to and from the pediatric clinic by themselves (without Vicki), then Junior would likely receive more attention. Thus, by choosing to work on behavioral controls, the nurse was stimulating change at several levels: whole-family system, parent-child subsystem, and marital/parental subsystem.

Review the Calgary Family Intervention Model

The nurse reviews the CFIM to stimulate her ideas about change and match interventions to the particular domain of family functioning: cognitive, affective, or behavioral. As we know from our own clinical practice, some interventions work better with some families than with others. It is desirable to address the specificity question; that is, "What intervention will most effect change with this particular problem with this particular family at this particular time?"

We encourage nurses to review CFIM, the intersection of domains of family functioning and intervention (Table 8–6), prior to deciding on a specific intervention or group of interventions. We have found in our own clinical work that sometimes we are biased toward one particular domain of family functioning (e.g., cognitive or affective) and thus are most likely (as a result of our own biases) to choose certain interventions whether or not they match the family's style of relating. Thus, we review the following before choosing a particular intervention for a particular family situation:

TABLE 8–6 CFIM: INTERSECTION OF DOMAINS OF FAMILY FUNCTIONING
AND INTERVENTIONS

		Interventions Offered by Nurse
Domains of Family Functioning	**Cognitive**	"**Fit**" **or Effectiveness**
	Affective	
	Behavioral	

- Questions as interventions
- Interventions directed at the cognitive domain of family functioning
- Interventions directed at the affective domain of family functioning
- Interventions directed at the behavioral domain of family functioning

When the nurse chooses interventions, we recommend that she choose ones that best match the problem that she and the family have agreed to change. The nurse and the Hamilton family agreed to meet for four sessions to learn how to manage Junior's behavior.

Another consideration in choosing an intervention is to pick one that flows from the nurse's hypothesis. Some interventions are more effective than others in bringing about change. One of the nurse's hypotheses with the Hamiltons was that Junior was negatively triangulated into the marital subsystem. Thus she decided to choose interventions that would establish a more firm marital boundary while at the same time promoting effective parental controls of Junior's behavior.

A further consideration in choosing interventions is to find ones that match the family's strengths. We believe that families have tremendous resources to solve their own problems and that intervention by outsiders should be kept to a minimum. The nurse, in working with the Hamiltons, was aware of their belief about themselves as "special." They took pride in the fact that they were "survivors" and had overcome such adversity as unemployment following a serious motor vehicle accident. The nurse decided to build on such strengths in developing the intervention plan.

A final consideration when choosing interventions is to pick ones that match the nurse's competence level. We have discussed in Chapters 5 and 7 ideas for the nurse to consider when evaluating her own competence level.

Choose Interventions

The following is a sample intervention plan for the Hamilton family.
Problem: Parent-Child System: Difficulty with Behavioral Control. The nurse decided to have a meeting with Mr. and Mrs.

Hamilton to discuss normal $3^{1}/_{2}$-year-old child behavior, how to set limits, and how to positively reinforce good behavior. The nurse chose interventions aimed at the following domains:

Cognitive Domain. The nurse thought of recommending books to the parents on behavior management skills if they were interested in reading on this topic.

Behavioral Domain. The nurse thought about asking the couple to gather information about the available child-management courses sponsored by local community agencies (e.g., school board, parent-teacher groups, day-care centers, and so forth).

Affective and Behavioral Domain. The nurse decided to invite Mr. Hamilton and Junior to a session with the hope of increasing positive feedback and attachment between them. Mrs. Hamilton and the nurse planned to sit behind a one-way mirror and coach Mr. Hamilton in improving his behavior management skills with Junior. Vicki would be left at the grandparents' home during this session. In this way, the nurse hoped to draw forth more positive experiences of unique outcomes for father and son and mother. At the same time, the nurse hoped that the grandparents, by babysitting Vicki, would be supportive of Mr. and Mrs. Hamilton but not critical of their parenting abilities.

Use of Questions as Interventions. Every time the nurse met with the Hamiltons, she asked *difference questions* that invited the family to comment on the differences between their past, present, and future behavior management skills. She also used *behavioral-effect questions* to stimulate more solution-focused conversation about the positive effects of appropriate behavioral control of Junior. That is, when Junior responded to the parents' appropriate behavioral limits, the nurse hoped the parents would recognize this.

We wish to emphasize that the nurse could have devised many other intervention plans to deal with the Hamilton's difficulty with behavioral control of Junior. For example, the nurse could have decided to focus more specifically on teaching the parents to control Junior's eating patterns. Had the nurse chosen to do this, she might then have invited Mrs. Hamilton to meetings to discuss nutrition for a $3^{1}/_{2}$-year-old child. During such sessions, the nurse would provide support for the mother. There is the danger, however, that the nurse, by having interviews only with the mother, might assume the role of "surrogate husband." The nurse would then exacerbate the difficulty between the husband and wife. This type of intervention would not match the nurse's hypothesis, although it could conceivably match the contracted problem. Instead of choosing to work only with the mother, the nurse elected to work with both parents. In this way, she was choosing an intervention consistent with her hypothesis and hoped to exert maximum leverage on the "problem-determined system."

HOW TO RECORD PROGRESS NOTES

After the nurse has developed an intervention plan and has continued to have contact with the family, she must maintain a record of the evolution of her work with the family. In particular, it is important for the specific work around the contracted presenting problem to be recorded. The ideal progress note provides a structure for the nurse to identify her hypothesis, connect the assessment and intervention components, and maintain a sense of the evolving nature of her work with the family through time. Most hospital and agency progress notes are blank sheets of

Family name: _____ Interview date: _____
Participants: _____ Interview place: _____
Nurse interviewer name and signature: _____

Hypothesis or plan preinterview:

New information:

Content/process of interview (including interventions and family's responses):

New hypothesis:

Plan for next meeting:

Figure 8–3. Sample progress note.

paper. They are not easily conducive to stimulating the nurse to connect her hypothesis with the assessment and intervention plan, never mind providing an opportunity for her to connect the family's responses to the intervention.

As shown on Figure 8–3, we have found the following areas helpful to address when writing progress notes:

1. We note the family members and the professionals who were present at the meeting, as well as the date and place of the meeting. This is particularly important if the interview takes place in a hospital setting, as frequently more professionals may be involved than just the nurse interviewer.
2. We record our hypotheses or plan for the interview prior to the meeting with the family. We have found this to be invaluable in focusing ourselves for the meeting. It does not mean that we are slaves to or become married to the plan. For example, if the family comes in with a new crisis, we can alter the plan, but it does mean that we have an idea of how we will approach the meeting prior to the interview.
3. We record the new information that the family tells us has happened since their last meeting. We are most interested in new information pertaining to changes in interaction around the presenting problem. These changes could be at the cognitive, affective, or behavioral domains of family functioning. For example, with the Hamilton family, the nurse recorded that the father reported he and his wife had gone to a parenting class the previous week. Following the class they had stopped for a quick meal, which he said was "the first time we were out together in 6 months without the children."
4. We record the content and process of the meeting. We include the interventions and the family's responses to them. For example, the nurse used future-hypothetical questions to follow up on the information that Mr. Hamilton reported about their going to the parenting class and out for a meal. The nurse asked the couple, "If you were to continue having time for yourselves to focus on parenting issues, what effect might this have on Junior's behavior?" The parents' response that they thought Junior would continue to be more compliant with them was recorded by the nurse.
5. We record a new hypothesis or a refinement of an old one. For example, as the Hamiltons progressed in achieving their goals, the nurse abandoned her hypothesis that the children were triangulated into the marriage. Rather, she developed a new hypothesis that focused on their strengths. She integrated the couple's previous history of positive coping (with the effects of a motor vehicle accident) and their need to deal with the effects of Junior's health problems (delayed speech and short stature).

6. We address the plan for the next meeting. We jot down any ideas that we have for the next meeting and aim to review them just prior to when we meet with the family.

When learning how to work with families, it is important for nurses to conceptualize problems within a systems framework. Learning both the "thinking" and "doing" can be facilitated by an integrated approach to record keeping (Bernstein & Burge, 1988). The progress note presented in this chapter structures interview recording in a manner that facilitates systems thinking. It reflects the evolving connections between assessment and intervention. Hypothesizing, session planning, intervention, and family response are inextricably connected. The nurse reviews the previous hypotheses, questions, content and process themes, interventions, and family responses prior to each meeting with the family. By carefully recording the evolution of the therapeutic conversation, the nurse is more likely to remain focused on change in the presenting problem. This effectively leads toward closure with the family.

How to Record a Discharge Summary

Some nurses, particularly those in community health settings, have an opportunity to synthesize their work with families by doing a discharge summary. Other nurses, particularly those in hospital settings, have less of an opportunity to synthesize, in a written manner, their work with families. Nevertheless, we believe that the opportunity to synthesize information into a termination summary is a useful and meaningful event for both the family and the nurse. We highly recommend that nurses take advantage of this opportunity. There are many ways one can record a discharge summary. In Chapter 4, we presented examples of some closing letters to families. In our own clinical work we have found the following areas useful to include in a discharge synopsis (Fig. 8–4):

1. We include the presenting problem and referral route information in one or two sentences. We find that this focuses the report so that all the information written is relevant to the identified problem.
2. We focus on the interventions used and the outcome. By identifying the interventions used, we are able to learn more about what worked and what did not work to effect change in the presenting issue. For example, in working with the Hamilton family, the nurse had recommended that the couple read books about effective behavioral management of children. She found that this intervention triggered a limited amount of change as neither the husband nor the wife was very interested in reading the material. Rather, they did benefit from the intervention in which the nurse asked them to "poll their friends, work colleagues, and relatives" about effective behavioral management strategies for young

Family name: _____ Date of first meeting: _____

Nurse's name: _____ Date of last meeting: _____

Nurse's signature: _____ Number of meetings: _____

Presenting problem and referal route:

Interventions and outcome:

Prognosis and recommendations:

Figure 8–4. Sample discharge summary.

children. The couple enjoyed "survey research" and found time to discuss the results together. They reported that they enjoyed discarding some of the ideas. However, they retained and used the ones that were most consistent with their own childrearing beliefs.

3. We address the area of prognosis and recommendations. Given the limited resources in our healthcare delivery systems, we find it useful to make recommendations that may be helpful if the family should re-present for additional assistance. For example, the nurse who worked with the Hamilton family recommended that if they should

ever need assistance in the future, it would be useful to inquire what was most useful and least useful about this series of contacts with the pediatric clinic. In the future, the nurse most likely would not try to use bibliotherapy as an intervention without reassessing with the family whether this type of intervention is one that might be useful. Rather, the nurse might recommend that experiments be tried by the couple in soliciting others' ideas about how to handle the new issue. Once having done that, the couple could then come back and discuss with the nurse the advantages and disadvantages of adopting these solutions. By recommending such ideas, the nurse builds on the information that she has gathered in working with the family this time. It does not prevent the new nurse interviewer from trying different ideas; it merely provides a tentative guide.

ISSUES IN RECORDING, STORING, AND ACCESSING RECORDS

Nurses are continually faced with issues about confidentiality. Who should have access to the family assessment summary or the discharge synopsis? Is it a family record or an individual record? Which family members can legally give consent for its release to another agency? Can the nurse talk to one family member about a meeting with another member when the first member is not present? These issues of confidentiality are becoming more numerous with the spread of communications technology. Family members sometimes request videotapes of their meetings so that they can play them on their own machines at home.

In the last decade, the subjects of human rights and confidentiality have increasingly come to the fore. In the areas of record content, release, consumer access, informed consent, records of minors, and compulsory reporting, nurses and other professionals have become increasingly more knowledgeable.

Guidelines regarding confidentiality exist in federal, state, and provincial regulations. Hospitals, clinics, and agencies also have guidelines for specialty areas. In the area of mental health, there is a great variety of age designation and conditions under which minors, for example, may receive care.

In family interviewing, confidentiality is a particularly complex issue. Data concerning more than one person are included in the file. Some of the family members are usually minors while some are adults. When children and adults are in treatment as a unit, care must be taken to protect the privacy of each person. Nurses would do well to be acquainted with their agency's or hospital's policies on confidentiality of family records.

Another practical issue concerning confidentiality is often raised. Family members sometimes try to obtain special attention by making telephone calls between sessions or by asking for private meetings with the nurse. The meaning of such behaviors should be carefully considered in the context of the nurse's understanding of the family system. For example, a nurse may be working with a family whose 25-year-old son is manic-depressive. The father, mother, and son may agree during a family interview that the young man should take lithium. If, however, the father calls the nurse after the family session to discuss why he believes his son should *not* take lithium, then the nurse should hypothesize about the meaning of the father's call. Could he fear disagreeing with his wife and son in front of them? Could he want the nurse to align with him against his wife and son? Generally, we recommend that nurses tell family members who request a private session that they bring their concerns to the family interviews. In this way, the nurse avoids becoming triangulated between two or more family members.

CONCLUSIONS

A particular format has now evolved in the process of family interviewing. The nurse ascertains whether a family assessment is indicated. If it is indicated, a family assessment is conducted. After the nurse has assessed the family, we recommend that the nurse review the CFAM categories and delineate a strengths/problems list. The nurse should then write a family assessment summary. A decision to intervene is based on a consideration of the family's level of functioning, the nurse's competence, and the work context. If intervention is indicated, then the nurse has to decide, in collaboration with the family, which are the key issues to focus on and which are tangential ones. We recommend that the nurse review the CFIM. The nurse must also consider which family members are to be seen and what is the frequency and length of treatment. An intervention plan should then be devised. The decision as to which interventions will be used to facilitate change within this particular family is a critical one. The nurse then records on a progress note a record of her therapeutic conversations with the family, and at the time of discharge synthesizes the work in a discharge summary.

REFERENCES

Bernstein, R., & Burge, S. (1988). A record-keeping format for training systemic therapists. *Family Process, 27*, 339–349.

Otto, H. (1963). Criteria for assessing family strength. *Family Process, 2*, 329–338.

Thorne, S., & Robinson, C. (1989). Guarded alliance: Health care relationships in chronic illness. *Image, 21*(3), 153–157.

HOW TO TERMINATE
WITH FAMILIES

To end professional contact with families in a way that is therapeutic is perhaps one of the most challenging aspects of the family interviewing process for nurses. Termination has been the least examined of the treatment phases in clinical work with families (Roberts, 1992). An important aspect of the termination stage is not only to end the nurse-family relationship therapeutically but also to do so in a manner that will sustain the progress that has been made. Nurses often establish very intense and meaningful relationships with families, and therefore may feel guilty or fearful about initiating termination. This chapter reviews the process of termination by examining the decision to terminate when it is initiated by the family, by the nurse, or as a result of the context in which the family finds themselves. Often the nurse's decision to terminate with a family does not necessarily mean that the family will cease contact with all professionals. Therefore, we discuss the process of referring families to other healthcare professionals. Specific suggestions for how to phase out and conclude treatment are given, as well as for how to evaluate the effects of the treatment process.

DECISION TO TERMINATE

NURSE-INITIATED TERMINATION

It is important to emphasize that it is not necessary that a total "cure" or complete resolution of the presenting problem or of all problems in the family be evident. Rather, it is the family's ability to master or to live with problems, not to eliminate them, that is the most important indicator for the decision to initiate termination. The termination stage evolves easily if the beginning and middle stages of treatment have concluded successfully. However, the most difficult decision for any nurse to make with regard to termination is the question of time. *When* is it the right time for termination? The question of when one should begin to think about termination boils down to what new solutions have been discovered to resolve old problems. If new solutions have been found and consequently the family functions differently, then that is the time to terminate because significant change has occurred. The skills necessary for nurse-initiated termination are given in a later section of this chapter (Phasing-out and Concluding Treatment) and in Chapter 5.

We have found the following ideas clinically useful in our own work when we have decided that additional meetings are not necessary and the family agrees. de Shazer (1982) recommends that families expand their perspective to include a focus on the positive behaviors rather than an exclusive focus on troublesome behaviors. Family members may be asked to record either mentally or on paper their observations of positive exceptions to the problem.

Another useful idea is one generated by White and Epston (1990), in which they recommend that the interviewer "expand the audience" to describe and acknowledge the family's unique outcomes and progress. For example, we often ask a family to tell us what advice they would have for other families confronting similar health problems. Sometimes, we have families write letters to other families to offer their suggestions of what has or has not worked in coping with a particular illness. One woman who had MS, but was successfully living with her illness, wrote a letter to a young woman who was not yet as successful. The letter gave hope and encouragement to this young woman. The older woman expressed that writing the letter was a very "cathartic" experience for her. She also went on to say, "MS is still here, but it does not dominate our lives and occupies only a small space over in the corner. I did experience a minor flare-up after Christmas but it cleared quickly. I remain optimistic." The nurse details the family's ideas and advice as a way both of reinforcing their positive ideas and of generating useful information for other families. Thus the family's competence is overtly acknowledged.

Lewis (1989) also suggests that the family be asked to pay close attention to *temporary* issues that may develop once the original problem has been managed adequately by the family. By describing such new issues as temporary and predictable reactions to the resolved original complaint, the nurse can prepare the family to visualize their issues as "daily living problems" rather than crises.

Termination rituals can also give family members courage to live their lives without the involvement of healthcare professionals (Roberts, 1992). If the initial concerns have been with children, we will often have a party—with balloons, cake, and all—to celebrate a child's mastering a particular problem such as enuresis. In addition, the child is given a certificate that says she or he has overcome the problem, whether it be enuresis, fighting fears, or putting chronic pain in its place.

Other families have been given something by the nursing team to symbolize their progress. For example, one family was given a feather to indicate that their problems now only require "the touch of a feather" to be able to keep them in place. It is essential to mark family strengths and problem-solving capabilities as families fully integrate back into their daily lives (Roberts, 1992) without the involvement of nurses.

FAMILY-INITIATED TERMINATION

When a family takes the initiative to terminate, it is very important for the nurse to acknowledge this and then to gain more explicit information regarding the family's reasons for wanting to terminate. This information will help the nurse to understand the family's responses to the interviewing process. For example, has the family discovered new solutions to their problems? Are the family and nurse able to identify and agree on significant changes that have occurred in individual and family functioning? Is the family also aware of how to sustain these changes? Segal (1991), in discussing the Brief Therapy approach of the Mental Research Institute, Palo Alto, California, suggests three criteria in the client's, or family's, report that indicates readiness to terminate. These three criteria are (1) a small, but significant, change has been made in the problem; (2) the change appears to be durable; and (3) the client/family implies or states an ability to handle things without the therapist.

If the family members specifically state that they wish to terminate, but the nurse believes this would be premature, then it is important for the nurse to take the initiative to review the family's decision. In so doing, the nurse reconceptualizes the progress that has been made by the family and recognizes what problems remain and what goals and solutions might yet be achieved. One way to do this is to have family members discuss with one another their desire to continue or discontinue sessions and to explore who is most in favor of which opinion. Also, the specifics of the decision may be helpful, such as when the family decided and what prompted them to decide on termination. After establishing who is most keen to continue, the nurse can invite that family member to share with the other family members the anticipated benefit of further sessions. It is helpful for families to be specific and emphasize the benefits that could be achieved if family interviewing were to continue. However, there are times when termination is inevitable. At such a point, it is reasonable and ethical for the nurse to accept the family's initiative to terminate and to do so without applying undue pressure, even though the nurse may disagree with their decision (Tomm & Wright, 1979).

We strongly urge nurses not to blame either families or themselves when they believe that families have prematurely left treatment. Rather, we encourage nurses to hypothesize about the factors that may have contributed to the termination. These factors may include such nurse behaviors as being too aligned with children, too slow to intervene, and so forth. Family behaviors such as involvement with other agencies and so forth also should be considered.

There are times, however, when family members state that they want to continue treatment, but they initiate termination indirectly. Indications of this may be late arrivals for the sessions, missed appointments, and the absence from sessions of family members who were specifically requested to attend (Barker, 1981). Another indicator that families are perhaps considering termination is when they express their dissatisfaction with the course of treatment or complain about the logistical difficulties of attending or the loss of time from work. We suggest that the same steps be taken as when the family initiates termination directly.

The challenge of family-initiated terminations is to determine if they are premature or not. In the nursing literature, there is a dearth of research to provide insights into reasons for premature terminations. However, the family therapy literature does have a few studies that suggest some of the reasons for premature termination by families. Gaines and Stedman (1981) evaluated 97 families over a 4-month period in a mental health clinic. They found that families who missed the first treatment session are at high risk to drop out over the course of treatment. The implication of missed appointments refers back to the importance of the engagement stage and even to the initial contact with families on the telephone.

In that same study, they discovered that failure of the family to bring all members to the first session (when the entire family was requested) is also a poor prognostic sign. Another interesting finding was that the nature of the referral source had a direct correlation with the family's continuing in treatment. Families who were referred by institutions (e.g., school, court) tended to discontinue treatment more frequently before achieving treatment goals than families who were individually referred (e.g., physicians, mental health professionals). The highest rate of continuation in treatment belonged to those who were self-referred.

A relationship between families with chronic problems and attendance in therapy was also found (Gaines & Stedman, 1981). Families with chronic problems attended more treatment sessions than families with acute problems, but they more frequently discontinued treatment before the treatment goals were reached.

Guldner (1981) also emphasized the importance of helping the family to understand the nature of the treatment contract. He suggested that many families have no real understanding of what should take place in family interviewing. Therefore, they may relate to the nurse as they do to physicians or clergy; they use the services as they wish and discontinue when they so desire.

CONTEXT-INITIATED TERMINATION

In some settings, particularly managed healthcare systems, it is not the nurse who initiates termination, but rather, closure is initiated by the healthcare system or insurance company. Ideally, some continued contact would be possible if family needs remained the same. In these situations, it is very important for the nurse to assess whether the family needs further treatment or whether it can continue to resolve problems and discover solutions on its own. If the family needs to be referred, the nurse requires some specific skills in this area. This process is discussed later in this chapter in the section entitled Referral to Other Professionals.

PHASING-OUT AND CONCLUDING TREATMENT

In Chapter 5, we highlighted some of the specific skills required for therapeutic termination in the form of learning objectives. We will now expand on these particular skills.

REVIEW CONTRACTS

We strongly encourage periodic review of the present status of the family's problems and changes. The use of a contract for a specific number of sessions provides a built-in way not only to set a time limit to the meetings but also to ensure periodic review. The contract also assists the nurse-interviewer in being mindful of the progress and direction of her work with families rather than seeing them as endless and without purpose beyond the vague good intention of "helping." We prefer a designated number of sessions to open-ended sessions. However, nurses need to be flexible as to the frequency and duration of sessions. Normally, the frequency decreases as problems improve. Periodic reviews allow family members to have the opportunity to express their pleasure or displeasure with the progress that is being made.

DECREASE FREQUENCY OF SESSIONS

If adequate progress has been made, then this is an ideal time to begin to decrease the frequency of sessions. In our experience, we have found that families are able to work toward termination more readily and with more confidence when they recognize the improvement in their own ability to solve problems (Tomm & Wright, 1979). Many families, however, find it difficult to acknowledge changes. In these circumstances, Tomm and Wright (1979) suggest the use of a question such as, "What would each of you have to do to bring the problem back?" to elicit a more explicit understanding or statement from family members regarding the changes that have been made.

Another very significant time to decrease the frequency of sessions is when the nurse has inadvertently fostered undue dependency. We have had many family situations presented to us in which nursing students or professional nurses provide "paid friendship" to mothers. These nurses have become the mother's major support system because they have not mobilized other supports such as husbands, friends, or relatives. In situations in which this dependency has occurred and is recognized, we strongly suggest that the nurse help foster other supports for the family and decrease the frequency of sessions.

If a nurse encounters hesitancy or reluctance to decrease the frequency of sessions or to terminate completely, the nurse should encourage a discussion of the fears related to termination and solicit support from other family members (Tomm & Wright, 1979). It has been our experience that family members frequently fear that if there are fewer sessions or if sessions are discontinued, they will not be able to cope with their problems or their problems will become worse. Thus, asking a question such as, "What are you most concerned would happen if we discontinued sessions now?" can get to the core of the matter very quickly. By clarifying family members' fears openly, other family members (who may be less fearful) have an opportunity to provide support.

GIVE CREDIT FOR CHANGE

Nurses have frequently chosen the profession of nursing because they have a strong desire to be helpful to individuals and families in obtaining optimal health. Their efforts are usually helpful, and they are often given all or much of the credit for changes and improvements. However, it has been our experience in family work that it is vitally important that the *family* receive the credit for change. There are several reasons for this necessity of stressing to the family that they are responsible for the change:

1. Families experience the tension, conflict, and anxiety of working through problems and, thus, families deserve the credit for improvement.
2. If the identified patient is a child and the nurse accepts credit, the nurse can be seen to be in a competitive relationship with the parents.
3. Perhaps the most important reason for giving the family credit for change is that this increases the chance that the positive effects of treatment will last. Otherwise, you may inadvertently convey the message that the family cannot manage without you and they will become indebted or too dependent. Termination provides an opportune time to comment on the positive changes that have already happened during the course of treatment.
4. Praising the family for its accomplishments in having helped or corrected the original presenting problem provides them with confidence in handling future problems. Specific statements such as, "You did the work" or "You are being far too modest" can reinforce to the family members that their efforts were essential in making the change.

It is never possible to really know what precipitated, perturbed, or initiated the change that occurs within families. Oftentimes, nurses create a context for change by assisting family members to explore intervention alternatives. Sometimes the very effort of bringing a family together in a room to discuss important family concerns can be the most significant intervention.

If families present themselves at termination with concerns about progress, we must express our appreciation for their positive efforts to solve problems constructively even when there has been no significant improvement. When such is the case, we strongly recommend that nurses discuss with their clinical supervisors some hypotheses of why the interview sessions do not seem to have been effective. Perhaps the goals of the family or the nurse have been too high or demanding. If the family does not progress, this is usually due to our inability to discover an intervention that is a fit with the family. Too often, we excuse ourselves from making further efforts to intervene when we label families as noncompliant, unmotivated, or resistant (Wright & Levac, 1992). It is very important, however, that the nurse believe that the family has worked hard despite minimal progress, and it is important to praise them for having done so.

We do not mean to imply, however, that because we are encouraging nurses to give families the credit for change that the nurse cannot enjoy the change. Family work can be very rewarding and certainly the nurse is part of the change process.

Evaluate Family Interviews

It is important to provide a formal closure to the end of the treatment process, with a face-to-face discussion whenever possible. During this final session, it is very valuable to evaluate the effectiveness of the treatment process and the effect of changes on various family members. Gurman and Kniskern (1981) recommend evaluating the impact not only on the whole family system but also on various subsystems, such as the marital subsystem and individual family-member functions. Such questions as, "What have you learned about yourself and MS?" and "What have you come to appreciate about your marriage?" invite reflection from the family about its changes. We also suggest asking family members the following questions: "What things did you find most/least helpful during our work together?" and "What things did you wish or were hoping would happen during our work together but did not?" In this way, the nurse demonstrates that she is also open and receptive to feedback. It is important at this time that the nurse not become defensive to any of the feedback but rather express appreciation to the family and inform them that this will assist the nurse and help in work with future families, which it will.

Extend an Invitation for Follow-up

Nurses often place themselves or are placed in situations known as "follow-up." However, the follow-up is often a negative experience for both the nurse and the family. For example, CHNs have reported that they are frequently requested to "check" on family members to assess their functioning. However, those who request the visit (e.g., a physician, the Department of Child Welfare) have made no clear statement to the family about the purpose of the visit. Therefore, the nurse is in a very awkward position. We strongly discourage nurses from placing themselves in these kinds of situations unless there has been clear, direct communication with the family by the requesting party. This type of follow-up, unfortunately, can give the message to the family that we anticipate further problems. It is better to make clear to the family that progress has been made and that the sessions are finished. However, you can let them know that if they would like input again in the future, you would be willing to see them. Families usually appreciate the availability of back-up support by professionals as resources in times of stress (Tomm & Wright, 1979).

For nurses employed in hospitals, the follow-up session always may not be possible. However, our experience has been that families do appreciate knowing if they will have future contact with the nurse who has worked intimately with them.

CLOSING LETTERS

Another way to positively punctuate the end of treatment is to send the family a letter giving a summary of the family sessions. This letter provides the opportunity to reinforce the changes made, plus offer the family members a review of their efforts and what they have accomplished. At the Family Nursing Unit (FNU), University of Calgary, closing letters are routinely sent to each family on completion of treatment. Many families have commented on how much they appreciate the letters and how they frequently refer back to them. An example of an actual closing letter follows. The names of the family members have been changed for purposes of confidentiality.

> Dear Family Barbosa:
>   Greetings from the Family Nursing Unit. We had the opportunity to meet with various members of your family on eight occasions. I have also had several phone conversations with both Venicio and Fatima in recent months.
>
> *Clinical Impressions:* Throughout our work together, our clinical nursing team has been very impressed with your family. Although a great many challenges have been presented to all of you over the past years, your family was able to overcome many obstacles and search for ways of helping each other through these difficult times.
>
> *What Our Team Learned from Your Family:* Our experience with your family has taught our clinical nursing team a great deal. The following is a synthesis:
>
> 1. Families dealing with a life-shortening illness with one of its members have the strength to deal with unresolved issues of blame, guilt, and shame. Even though there has been a great deal of pain and hurt in a family, they can heal their relationships and move on.
> 2. Although it can be a common response for family members to distance themselves from the possibility of death with a life-shortening illness and to be afraid of dying, it is possible for family

members to make peace with each other and find peace in themselves, giving them the courage to go on.

3. Even though a mother and son may reside in different places and may not see each other that often, they can still play a significant part in each other's lives. No matter how old a child and parent are, the knowledge that they love and accept each other for what they are can make a significant difference in their lives.

4. The uncertainty involved with a life-shortening illness can be the most difficult thing for families to handle. Family members can help each other with the uncertainty by discussing the situation openly amongst themselves.

5. Grandparents and grandsons have very special relationships that are different from parents and sons.

As you all continue to face the many challenges that are ahead, we trust that you will draw upon your own special strengths as well as on more open communication to help you meet these challenges. It was truly a privilege to work with you. We wish you continued strength for the future.

Should you desire further consultation at any time, you can arrange this with the Family Nursing Unit's secretary, Marlene Baier. A Research Assistant will be in contact with you in approximately six months to ask you to participate in our outcome study to ascertain your satisfaction with the Family Nursing Unit.

Sincerely,

Jane Nagy, RN, BN   Lorraine M. Wright, RN, PhD
Masters Student   Director, Family Nursing Unit
                             Professor, Faculty of Nursing

Therapeutic letters, whether sent during clinical work with families or at the end of treatment, have proven to be a very useful and often potent intervention to invite families to reflect on ideas offered within the session, as well as to reflect on changes they have made over the course of sessions (Watson & Lee, 1992; White & Epston, 1990; Wright & Nagy, 1993; Wright & Simpson, 1991; Wright & Watson, 1988).

REFERRAL TO OTHER PROFESSIONALS

Referrals to other professionals may be advisable for a variety of reasons. We will list some specific tasks that are required to make a smooth transition for the family from one professional to another. First, however, we will discuss some of the more common reasons for nurses to refer families to other professionals.

With the expanding specialty areas within nursing, it is becoming impossible and totally unrealistic to expect that nurses can be experts in all areas. Therefore, there are times when it is most appropriate for nurses to seek the input of additional professional resources when problems are quite complex. A nurse may refer families or specific family members for consultation or ongoing treatment. For example, if a senior family member is experiencing temporal headaches, it is very important that any organic or biologic origin of this problem be ruled out. Therefore, a nurse might refer the family for consultation with a neurologist and may suspend treatment until the consultation is complete.

In other instances, the nurse may discover that a particular child has a learning disability and that this is out of the realm of the nurse's expertise. The nurse may suggest referring the child to an education center where they have greater expertise in dealing with children with learning difficulties. Nurses need to be open to referring individuals or entire families for consultation. It is inappropriate for nurses to perceive this as an inadequacy in their own repertoire of skills. In order to refer wisely, nurses need to have an extensive knowledge of professional resources within the community.

Another reason for referring to other professionals, but not as common as the one above, is if the family moves or is transferred to another setting. If the family moves, is transferred, or is discharged before treatment is over, it is very important that the nurse, especially in a hospital setting, maximize the opportunities to do family work (Wright & Bell, 1981). A beautiful illustration of this was given by one of our graduate nursing students. Following some university seminars on the importance of family interviewing, this student, who was working part-time in a rural hospital, invited the parents of an asthmatic child to a family interview. The student obtained much valuable information regarding the interrelationship of the child's asthmatic problem with other family dynamics. Shortly thereafter, the child was discharged. The nursing student ascertained that the family was interested in changing the recurring problem of frequent admissions for this young child. The student made an appropriate referral to the mental health services within the community. This highlights the point that with only *one* family interview, an assessment can be made and a significant intervention completed through referral for a recurring problem.

Some of the specific tasks required to make appropriate referrals follow.

PREPARE FAMILIES

It is most important to prepare families adequately so that they understand the nature of the referral to a new professional. This can be done by explaining directly to families the reason for the referral and why the nurse feels they would benefit from it. Another method that can be useful for ensuring openness and clarity about the nature of the referral is for the nurse to write a summary and then to review this summary with the family. This summary can then be sent to the new professional and a copy made available for the family. In this way, the family is not left wondering what information will be shared with the new professional. Also, an important implicit message is given that this information is confidential and private *about them* and, therefore, they have a right to know what is shared.

Selecting a new professional can sometimes pose a challenge. If a nurse is known in the community, it is wise to solicit the help of colleagues for ideas and advice on which agencies or professionals are best for the type of treatment needed, or to seek information from community information directories and booklets.

Meet the New Professional

It has been our experience that the transition to the new professional is much more effective and efficient if the nurse can be present with the family at the first meeting. In this way, a more personal referral is made. It often reduces the fears and anxieties that families may have about starting "fresh" with someone new. Prior to the referral, opportunities should be given to the family to express concerns or ask questions about the referral. At the first meeting, the family may wish to clarify with the new professional what their expectations and understanding are of the referral. The new professional can also clarify her understanding of the reason for the referral and any misconceptions can be dealt with at that time. A conjoint meeting with the family, nurse, and new professional can also serve as a "marker" for the end of the nurse's relationship with the family.

Keep Appropriate Boundaries

When a family has been referred but the nurse continues to provide care for the family's physical needs, it is extremely important that boundaries of responsibility be clear. Otherwise, the nurse could inadvertently become triangulated between the family and the new professional.

For example, a home-care nurse regularly visited an elderly patient who lives with her adult daughter. The purpose of the visits by the home-care nurse was to assist with colostomy care. The nurse observed and assessed the interaction between the elderly parent and the adult daughter as a severe and long-standing conflict. This conflict was having a negative effect, deterring the elderly patient from assuming more responsibility for her physical care. Due to the nurse's family assessment skills, she was able to make an important referral to a family therapy program where more indepth work on the intergenerational conflict began. However, in future visits with the elderly patient, the nurse was listening to complaints about the adult daughter that the patient was not discussing in the family meetings. Also, the family therapist called the nurse and asked the nurse to apply pressure on the elderly parent to be more cooperative in attending sessions. Thus, very quickly the nurse had become "caught in the middle" between the family and the therapist. The nurse dealt with the situation by requesting to join in a meeting with the family and the therapist to clarify the expectations of all parties. In this one session, the nurse was able to "detriangulate" herself by clarifying her present role with the family and the new professional.

TRANSFERS

In our more than 20 years of clinical experience, we have not found the practice of transferring families from one nurse to another to be very successful. We view the process of transfers as very different from referrals. A referral is usually made to another healthcare professional with different expertise. A transfer, on the other hand, is usually made to another nursing colleague of similar expertise and competence. We recommend, if at all possible, that nurses conclude treatment with the families they are working with rather than transfer them to a colleague. In our experience, families frequently disengage from the new nurse through missed appointments, no-shows, or not stating any particular concern. It is understandable that families do not wish to "start over" with another nurse if at all possible. We hypothesize that transfers are frequently made to assuage the nurse's feelings about leaving versus the family's desires about continuing treatment.

SUCCESS OF TREATMENT IN FAMILY WORK

Although interventions may obtain positive and possibly dramatic results *during* treatment, the real success of family work is the positive changes that are *maintained* or continue to evolve weeks and months after nurses have terminated treatment with particular families. We strongly encourage professional nurses and nursing students to make it a pattern of practice to obtain data from the family as to outcome. When there is a focus on outcome, it directs the nurse to orient her work toward change, focus on problems that can be changed, and think of how the family will cope without the nurse in the future. We also suggest that in any follow-up with families, the nurse can explain that this is a *normal* pattern of practice (e.g., "We normally contact families with whom we have worked within six months to gain information on how things are evolving"). It is also important to use this follow-up with specific goals in mind. Thus, a very useful reason for follow-up can be for research purposes. In our experience, beginning nurse interviewers tend to be more focused on what is going on in the family, whereas more experienced nurses focus on quite specific goals for treatment. Carter (1986) also suggests that "the criteria for 'success' change over the course of a career, and that it is not so much one's view of success that changes as one's view of what is possible" (p. 19). Therefore, outcome is important.

To facilitate evaluation, we suggest formalizing follow-up of families either by live interview, questionnaire, or both. At present, we favor the use of a questionnaire that is answered by all available family members.

At the FNU, University of Calgary, families are routinely interviewed 6 months following the last session by a research assistant who has had no previous contact with the families (Wright, Watson, & Bell, 1990). This outcome study is designed to evaluate the services provided by the FNU. The variables examined by this study are the family's satisfaction with the services provided, satisfaction with the nurse interviewer, and change in the presenting problem and family relationships. An instrument designed for this study asks for each family member's perspective on each of the variables. Questions are asked in relation to two time periods: at the conclusion of the family sessions and at the time of the survey. Results from the survey (n=80) indicate that the most helpful aspects of family sessions were the opportunity to ventilate family concerns, thereby increasing communication among family members, and obtaining support from the FNU clinical nursing team. Families ranked the interview process and the suggestions from the FNU clinical nursing team as the second most helpful aspects (Wright et al., 1990).

Ninety-four percent of the family members reported satisfaction with the nurse interviewer, who was usually a Masters student specializing in family systems nursing. They indicated that the friendly, professional, and nonthreatening manner of the graduate nursing students made them comfortable.

More than 70 percent of the family members reported that the presenting problem was better at the time of the survey. This represents a 6 to 18 percent increase from the family members' initial reports of improvement in the presenting problem at the conclusion of the family sessions. Regardless of the presenting problem, 64.6 percent of fathers and 66.7 percent of mothers reported positive changes in the marital relationship, such as increased communication, improved relationships, and decreased tension, suggesting support for the systems theory tenet that change in one part of the system effects change in other parts (Wright et al. 1990).

This type of outcome study follows the advice of Gurman and Kniskern (1981), who suggest that assessing change should be evaluated at the individual, parent-child, marital, and family system levels. Gurman and Kniskern (1981) believe that a "higher level of positive change has occurred when improvement is evidenced in systemic (total family) or relationship (dyadic) interactions than when it is evidenced in individuals alone" (p. 765). "That is, individual change does not logically require system change, but stable system change does require individual change and relationship change, and relationship change requires individual changes" (p. 766).

Family treatment does appear to be having creditable success as reported by outcome studies in family therapy. However, nurses could contribute significantly to family outcome research by focusing on follow-up with families in which a particular family member experiences a health problem. This area of family work is just beginning to be researched and lends itself beautifully to the active involvement of nurses in its evolution.

CONCLUSIONS

In reading this chapter, it can be seen that the matter of concluding treatment in a therapeutic and constructive way is a challenge for any nurse working with families. Unfortunately, much more has been written in the literature about how to begin with and treat families than about how to terminate with them. However, we want to emphasize the extreme importance of terminating contact with families in a manner that will increase the likelihood of change being maintained and even expanded.

REFERENCES

Barker, P. (1981). *Basic family therapy*. Baltimore: University Park Press.

Beck, M. (1981). Therapist-initiated termination from family therapy. *American Journal of Family Therapy, 9*, 94–95.

Carter, B. (1986, July/August). Success in family therapy. *Family Therapy Networker, 10*, 17–22.

de Shazer, S. (1982). *Patterns of brief family therapy: An ecosystemic approach.* New York: Guilford Press.

Gaines, T., & Stedman, J. M. (1981). Factors associated with dropping out of child and family treatment. *American Journal of Family Therapy, 9*, 45–51.

Guldner, C. A. (1981). Premature termination in marital and family therapy. In A. S. Gurman (Ed.), *Questions and answers in the practice of family therapy* (pp. 510–512). New York: Brunner/Mazel.

Gurman, A. S., & Kniskern, D. P. (1981). Family therapy outcome research: Knowns and unknowns. In A. S. Gurman (Ed.), *Handbook of family therapy* (pp. 742–775). New York: Brunner/Mazel.

Lewis, W. (1989). How not to engage a family in therapy. *Journal of Strategic and Systemic Therapies, 8*(1), 50–53.

Roberts, J. (1992). Termination rituals. In T. S. Nelson & T. S. Trepper (Eds.), *101 Interventions in family therapy*. Binghamton, NY: Haworth Press.

Segal, L. (1991). Brief therapy: The MRI approach. In A. S. Gurman & D. P. Kniskern (Eds.), *Handbook of family therapy* (Vol. 2, pp. 171–199). New York: Brunner/Mazel.

Stanton, J. D. (1981). Who should get credit for change which occurs in therapy? In A. S. Gurman (Ed.), *Questions and answers in the practice of family therapy* (pp. 519–522). New York: Brunner/Mazel.

Tomm, K., & Wright, L. M. (1979). Training in family therapy: Perceptual, conceptual and executive skills. *Family Process, 18*, 227–250.

Watson, W. L., & Lee, D. (1993). Is there life after suicide? The systemic belief approach for "survivors" of suicide. *Archives of Psychiatric Nursing, 7*(1), 37–42.

White, M., & Epston, D. (1990). *Narrative means to therapeutic ends.* New York: W. W. Norton.

Wright, L. M., & Bell, J. (1981). Nurses, families and illness: A new combination. In D. S. Freeman & B. Trute (Eds.), *Treating families with special needs* (pp. 199–205). Ottawa: Canadian Association of Social Workers.

Wright, L. M., & Levac, A. M. (1992). The non-existence of non-compliant families: The influence of Humberto Maturana. *Journal of Advanced Nursing, 17*, 913–917.

Wright, L. M., & Nagy, J. (1993). Death: The most troublesome family secret of all. In E. Imber-Black (Ed.), *Secrets in families and family therapy* (pp. 121–137). New York: W. W. Norton.

Wright, L. M., & Simpson, P. (1991). A systemic belief approach to epileptic seizures: A case of being spellbound. *Contemporary Family Therapy: An International Journal, 13*(2), 165–180.

Wright, L. M., & Watson, W. L. (1988). Systemic family therapy and family development. In C. J. Falicov (Ed.), *Family transitions: Continuity and change over the life cycle* (pp. 407–430). New York: Guilford Press.

Wright, L. M., Watson, W. L., & Bell, J. M. (1990). The Family Nursing Unit: A unique integration of research, education and clinical practice. In J. M. Bell, W. L. Watson, & L. M. Wright (Eds.), *The cutting edge of family nursing* (pp. 95–109). Calgary, Alberta: Family Nursing Unit Publications.

INDEX

An "f" following a page number indicates a figure; a "t" indicates a table.